ESSE
OILS FOR
LIFE

by Shirly Line

foulsham
LONDON • NEW YORK • TORONTO • SYDNEY

Dedication

I dedicate this book to Ray Caylers who very sadly died this year. His energy and efficiency everybody who knew him appreciated — and especially for the support he gave me at all times.

foulsham
Yeovil Road, Slough, Berkshire SL1 4JH

ISBN 0-572-01808-8

Printed in Great Britain by Cox & Wyman Ltd, Reading, Berks.
Phototypeset in Great Britain by Typesetting Solutions, Berks.

CONTENTS

Foreword   4

Introduction   6

Chapter 1: Omega 3 Plus   11

Chapter 2: Helpful Hints   13

Chapter 3: Simple Sauces   16

Chapter 4: A — Z of Omega 3   22

Index   127

FOREWORD

If we in Europe eat more fish it will be beneficial to our health! It is now official! Researchers have known for the past 20 years that societies such as the Eskimos and Japanese which eat a lot of fish, have less coronary heart disease and cancers than western societies which consume less fish. Western researchers have concluded that we could derive the same benefits by increasing our fish consumption.

During the past 20 years, studies in Europe and the USA have measured the effect of increasing dietary fish and fish oil on a number of diseases. The results have been very favourable. Studies have demonstrated that increasing our fish consumption results in a decreased risk of heart disease and other vascular diseases. This benefit results from a lower risk of having 'heart attacks' and 'strokes', the two events which actually cause death in people suffering from arteriosclerosis.

Fish and fish-oil produce these beneficial effects, because they contain high levels of the important OMEGA 3 fatty acids. These are the 'building-blocks' for some very important tissue metabolites which control not only blood clotting, but also the development of arteriosclerosis, hypertension and chronic inflammation.

Western man has become 'deficient' in OMEGA 3 fatty acids. Many of the chronic diseases mentioned above could be reduced significantly by eating more Omega-3, THAT IS, BY EATING MORE FISH. The evidence is now so strong that many international bodies, such as the UK Nutrition Society, have published these findings stating clearly that OMEGA 3 fatty acids are essential for human health and that we should consume more of them.

It is therefore appropriate that this book on fish and shellfish should be published at this time. If the book succeeds in increasing consumption of fish, it will be doing a tremendous favour to individuals, health authorities and western society at large.

Dr Desmond A Rice MVB, MRCVS, Ph.D
Nutrition Services (Int) Ltd
N. Ireland

INTRODUCTION

About the Author

Shirly Line was born in Blackpool very close to the water and sands. This probably provided the genesis for her passion for the sea and everything in it. Helped by many childhood ventures spent fishing with her father off the Cornish coast (tied to the mast!), she has acquired a wealth of knowledge on cooking, writing, talking about and eating fish and shellfish. Although, she freely admits that it would take a lot longer than one lifetime to know all there is to know about her favourite subject!

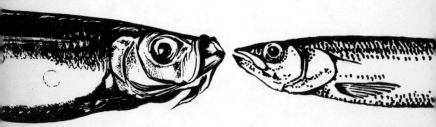

Shirly's interest in **OMEGA** 3 came about when the opportunity arose to work in Switzerland for several years. Doctors from Geneva University Hospital encouraged her to write a diabetic recipe book, in French. Their advice was to include plenty of fish and shellfish in the book, translate it back into English and go home and teach people to eat more seafood! Which she did.

A busy few years ensued, taking her from Radio 74 in

France to Scotland to Radio Kent, talking not only on the real benefits of fish and shellfish but also the value of 'real food' for better health.

Shirly's first cookbook, Cooking The New Diabetic Way, with Gill Metcalf was first published by Ward Lock in 1983. It is available in braille and calculated for the USA. She has two books being released in 1993; 101 Fishy Dishes Caught By Shirly Line, and New Nouvelle Cuisine For Diabetics, Family and Friends – plus Eat Plenty, Stay Fit and Thin.

Acknowledgements

I am truly grateful to my many friends in the 'fishy' business who have not only given me the inspiration, but also their time to make this little book possible. Without their advice and enthusiasm, so many people would be deprived of the knowledge on the value of fish and shellfish in the diet and how they can make for a healthier, and therefore better, quality of life.

I thank all my pals in Billingsgate Fish Market, who I have driven quite mad over the years with my 'how?', 'why?', and 'what for?', with a special thanks to Don Ruth, Billingsgate fish porter, Liveryman of The Worshipful Company of Fishmongers, London.

Thank you also: Dr. Eric Edwards, Director of The Shellfish Association of Great Britain for your support and advice — as always. Thank you Peter Davidson, Dengie Shellfish, Burnham-on-Crouch —I think we got it right.

Thank you to The Sea Fish Industry Authority for most of the super line drawings of popular species of fish and shellfish; not to forget John Early at Torry Research, and thank you to Michael, always on the end of my line to listen and help.

Doreen (Shellfish Association of Great Britain) and Ray Liberty — we coped with a few rush jobs in our time. Stephen Hall, for putting humour into so much of my work as a fellow diabetic. And a special thank you to Sue Payne.

Words of Inspiration

There is a wealth of nutritious and tasty natural food swimming around the world's oceans. That means plenty of fine fish and shellfish around our coasts, in our rivers, ponds and lochs, and from the ever increasing number of fish and shellfish farms. And it's all waiting to jump onto our plates, guaranteeing better health and extra brain food for both young and old alike.

This little book proves how easy it is to prepare and cook fish and shellfish — with none of the fancy sauces and complicated methods to camouflage and baffle those who say they 'can't cook'. It also advises on availability; no longer a problem for the housewife who lives under Banbury Cross, since many supermarkets now have decent fresh fish counters and freezer cabinets full of frozen seafood products.

I have included simple drawings for easy identification of fish and shellfish to help you when faced with that very stupendous display of colours, shapes and sizes on the fishmonger's slab. And without doubt I cover the most vital issue of the lot — fish for good health.

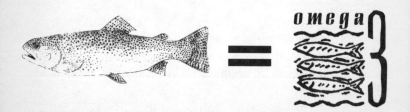

All fish and shellfish contain natural polyunsaturated oils that are recognized by the medical experts as being essential in the daily diet. Very technical and complicated names (that I defy anyone to pronounce) describe these essential fishy oils — EICOSAPENTAENOIC ACID (EPA) and DOCOSAHEXAENOIC ACID (DHA) — shall we just say OMEGA 3?

The Greenland Eskimos have one of the lowest rates of heart disease, diabetes and arthritis. They not only enjoy a staple diet of fish, they also indulge in plenty of fish blubber; which is very necessary to keep themselves warm.

The Japanese are the largest consumers of fish and shellfish throughout the whole world. They are quite paranoid about their consumption, so much so that they even have a daily newspaper relating solely to fish and shellfish. No wonder their brains are so big; perhaps the old wives tale 'fish is food for the brain' has a ring of truth after all!

● It is now a proven fact that OMEGA 3 will reduce the risks of heart disease and all related problems, including heart attack, stroke, high blood pressure, thrombosis and high cholesterol level in the blood. Shellfish was warned against by doctors in the past because of the minute cholesterol content; now oysters and scallops are said to offer more benefit than risk. Shellfish is back in medical favour!

While women are generally less prone to heart attacks, they are quite likely to catch up after the menopause. ● OMEGA 3 oils those arthritic joints and all allied 'creaky' conditions. ● Eczema, psoriasis, asthma, hay fever, migraine headaches, multiple sclerosis, diabetes, over-active thyroid and bowel ailments, like diverticulitis and colitis, can all be helped with a regular supply of OMEGA 3. ● Studies now show that OMEGA 3 may even prohibit the development of mammary, colonic and prostatic cancer.

Make no mistake, OMEGA 3 is not a miracle cure, but surely worth giving more than a second thought.

The body is unable to make OMEGA 3 for itself, so it must be provided for in the diet — a diet that contains a good supply of fish and shellfish. A minute amount of OMEGA 3 can be found in linseed oil and sea vegetables (sea weeds), but there is no other source of supply known to date (although you could take a fish oil capsule).

Halibut and orange capsules were allocated 'free gratis' by the government after World War II. Although we now have to pay for our OMEGA 3 (fish oil), one can hardly complain about the price of fresh or tinned sardines, pilchards, fresh or tinned mackerel and herrings or tinned tuna. We don't have to rely on a free capsule, and we don't have to rely on a daily helping of caviare, reputed to be one of the richest sources of OMEGA 3 in the world.

Farmed salmon and trout are almost cheaper to feed the family on than bacon and eggs! The Pacific (gigas) oyster could soon be rocking the salted peanut from its stool at the cocktail, tapas, cafe, bistro and pub counter — what bliss!

Keith Floyd has worked wonders around the world in putting fun back into the preparation and cooking of fish and shellfish — this is my effort at serious fun. OMEGA 3 will get through to father's heart, lubricate granny's creaky joints, give confidence to spotty teenagers, expectant mums; and 'Uncle Tom Cobbly and all'. Get into The Essential Fish-Oil Diet right now. You will be eating Seafood For Life itself.

Shirly Line 1993

Chapter 1

OMEGA 3 PLUS

It is not always the most expensive fish that provides the best nutritional value for good health — so it is no excuse to say that fish is too expensive! Eat fish twice or three times a week to keep fit — stay very fit by remembering that the fish and shellfish contained in the following list have the highest ratings of OMEGA 3.

Anchovies
Baracuda
Bonito – cousin of oily Tuna and Mackerel
Brisling – baby Sprat
Buckling – smoked Herring
Carp – plenty in Gefilte
Caviare – roe of Beluga, Oscietre or Sevruga
Cod Cheeks – from Cod
Roe (Coral) – of the Scallop
Garfish
Grayling
Greenland Halibut
Grey Mullet
Halibut – fresh or frozen
Huss — Dogfish or Rock Salmon
Herrings
Kingfish – big Mackerel

Kippers – smoked Herrings
Lamprey – loved in France
Lumpfish Roe
Mackerel
Marlin – cousin to Swordfish
Perch
Pilchards
Razor Fish
Red Mullet
Roach
Sardines – fresh or tinned
Sea Urchin
Shad – cousin to Herring
Sprat
Swordfish – usually frozen
Tench – popular in France
Trout – all species
Tuna – fresh or tinned
Whitebait – fresh or frozen

All recipes containing a very high content of OMEGA 3 are clearly marked with the **OMEGA 3 logo**.

Recognized Fish & Shellfish Caught in British Water

Sea Fish

Anchovy
Bass
Brill
Catfish
Cod or Codling
Coley (Saithe or Coalfish)
Conger Eel
Dab
Dogfish (Flake, Huss or Rigg)
Eel
Flounder
Garfish
Grey Mullet
Gurnard
Haddock
Hake
Halibut
Herring
John Dory
Ling
Mackerel
Megrim
Monkfish or Angler
Pilchard
Plaice
Pollack
Razor Fish
Red Mullet
Sardine
Sea Bream
Skate or Ray
Smelt
Sole, Dover or Lemon
Sprat
Turbot
Whitebait
Whiting
Witch

Freshwater Fish

Carp
Pike
Salmon
Brown Trout
Sea Trout
Rainbow Trout

Shellfish

Clam
Cockle
Crab
Crawfish
Crayfish
Lobster
Mussel
Oyster
Prawn
Sea Urchin
Shrimp, Pink or Brown
Scallop
Scampi (Norway Lobster or Dublin Bay Prawn
Squid
Whelk
Winkle

Chapter 2

HELPFUL HINTS

Fresh fish and shellfish are simple foods. Lengthy instructions in this little book on preparation and cooking aren't really necessary.

Sauces are only required to camouflage, impress or make a little go a long way.

Don't overcook fish; remember that a good amount of fish and shellfish can be enjoyed raw and tastes quite delicious.

If you can't afford smoked salmon try smoked mackerel — boneless kippers sliced with a squeeze of lemon are delectable.

Leftovers of fish mixed with leftover mashed or instant potatoes make a tasty meal for the kids — they love fish cakes with tomato sauce; a little chopped smoked fish gives grandpa a zing!

Groundnut oil is perfect for frying fish — don't be too penny-pinching and change the oil regularly. A little butter painted over less oily fish like cod, hake, turbot will do no harm to the cholesterol level. Fish loaded with OMEGA 3 needs no oil or butter when grilling, it has it's own built-in supply.

When coating fish or shellfish with flour for deep frying, pop the flour with seasoning into a plastic bag, add the fish or shellfish and give a little shake to cover evenly — easy! Alternatively, use oatmeal to coat fish when frying, just for a change.

Yogurt (low fat) or fromage frais (low fat) are a magic substitute for cholesterol laden rich cream.

And always make use of your Friendly Fishmonger, he loves to help out in filleting and beheading if need be — but don't let him keep the heads, bones and skin as they make a super fish stock.

The microwave is magic and has so many useful advantages, but be careful when cooking fresh fish and shellfish — they need so little cooking time. The exception is conger eel; this tough fella certainly needs 30 minutes to the 450g (1lb) in a fish stew or pie, unless cut into tiny pieces.

Freezing

Ideal if you are lucky enough to be presented with a big bag of 'freebies' by your friendly fishing enthusiast. But be warned, whatever you take out of the freezer, don't ruin the flavour completely by 'popping into boiling water for a quick thaw' — ruination! Always allow any frozen fish and shellfish to thaw to room temperature and never, ever, re-freeze.

Keeping Fish – Don't!

Get the fish or shellfish home and remove the wrapping as soon as possible, pop on a plate and cover with foil or cling-film, a cloth or a plate. Keep in the refrigerator until ready to cook. Eat within 24 hours.

Does Fish Smell – No!

There should be no strong smell if the fish or shellfish is really fresh. If fish and shellfish smells of ammonia —throw it away.

Sea Vegetables

Keep an eye alert for the farmed sea vegetables (commonly known as seaweed) that are now becoming popular in some supermarkets. Wakame, kombu and nori have been used for years in Japanese cooking — not only are they rich in minerals and vitamins but quite a few sea vegetables do contain our best friend, OMEGA 3. Crispy, dried dulse makes a change from salted peanuts, Irish carragheen is at last being recognized and laverbread with scallops is scrumptious. Add a little mystery and OMEGA 3 to your simple fish pie, add 25g (1oz) sea vegetables and keep the guests guessing.

Using Fresh Herbs

Any fresh herbs, rather than the packets of dried, will enhance a fish stew, soup or salad. Tarragon, parsley, fennel, dill and chives are wondeful, and mint is magic. Also remember, for the herb gardener who finds everything ready for picking on the same day in the year, fresh herbs freeze so you will have a fresh supply for the winter.

Saffron

Saffron is king of all the spices; and my very special sunshine from Spain. Christened 'Red Gold' by Roman and Persian emperors, who were the only privileged few allowed to indulge in this golden aromatic aphrodisiac, saffron is now available from Spain to all. Arabs from way back in the tenth century introduced the cultivation of this valuable spice into Spain, which has been valued greatly throughout the centuries. The unique technique of farming and processing La Mancha saffron has never been allowed to change in Spain. Hand planted, hand picked, hand packed – *precioso puro oro rojo.* For so many fish soups, stews and shellfish dishes, *Cefran* gold is essential; who can imagine a scrumptious paella without real Spanish saffron?

Chapter 3

SIMPLE SAUCES

Really fresh fish asks for nothing more than to be cooked 'with loving care' — not a long time. A sauce is not necessary, other than to make a little go a long way. If you are having a party — that's different. The following are my basic personal sauce choices for fish: if the occasion is right and I have the time.

Real mayonnaise must go with fresh cold salmon. If you follow the basic rules, you can't go wrong. If you really can't be bothered, do buy mayonnaise that is marked 'real mayonnaise made with eggs' — I do, frequently!

Wobbly Mayonnaise

Use one very, very, fresh egg yolk that has been out of the refrigerator for at least 2 hours. In a very clean bowl with an electric hand mixer, beat the yolk with ½ teaspoon Dijon mustard until creamy in colour. Measure 200ml (7fl oz/⅞ cup) good oil, sunflower or olive, into a jug and, with the mixer running, add the oil drip by drop by drip — very, very slowly. I know it may seem daft, but it should take about 4 minutes to add 8 drips of oil — if you work any faster the whole lot will curdle. After the first stage you can allow the oil to drip more quickly. Mix in a little lemon juice or wine vinegar when the mayonnaise is really thick, and add a little seasoning to taste.

Serve in a wine glass with lemon slices garnishing the

rim of the glass. Good with any cold fish — add a few drops of brandy when serving with large scampi or prawns.

Variations

Garlic Mayonnaise — to go with shellfish. Crush 5 cloves of garlic and mix into the mayonnaise.
Lemon Mayonnaise — perfect with cold white fish. Add juice and grated rind of a lemon to the mayonnaise.
Tartare Sauce — use with any flat fish. Add chopped gherkin, a few capers and a little lemon juice to the mayonnaise. A little sieved hard-boiled egg can also be added.

Lemon Sauce

Serves 4

Ingredients

	Metric	Imperial	American
cold pressed virgin olive oil	2 tbsp	2 tbsp	2 tbsp
flour	25 g	1 oz	¼ cup
juice of lemons	2	2	2
grated rind of lemon	1	1	1
fish stock made up with fish bones, head and skin, plus a few herbs	200 ml	7 fl oz	⅞ cup
pinch sea salt			
a little freshly ground black pepper			
egg yolk	1	1	1

Method

Make this sauce in an electric sauce maker if you have

one, or use a basin over a pan of hot water (bain marie). Blend the oil and flour over gentle heat. Add the lemon juice and rind with the stock and seasoning. Keep stirring and beat in the egg yolk — do not allow the mixture to boil otherwise it will curdle. Keep stirring until the sauce is creamy and thick. Really good with poached or grilled halibut and turbot.

Minty Cream Sauce

Mix a small carton of natural low-fat yogurt with 2 tablespoons mayonnaise and lots of chopped fresh mint — a squeeze of lemon juice and a little pepper can be added. Ideal for fish salads.

My Parsley Sauce

Serves 4

Ingredients

	Metric	Imperial	American
butter	25 g	1 oz	2 tbsp
flour	1 tbsp	1 tbsp	1 tbsp
skimmed milk	300 ml	½ pint	1¼ cups
fresh parsley, chopped	25 g	1 oz	1 oz
egg, beaten	1	1	1

Method

Melt the butter in a pan. Blend in the flour over a low heat until smooth. Gradually add the milk, stirring continuously to make a smooth sauce. Add the parsley and egg, stir for a further few minutes over a low heat. Keep warm in a serving dish over a pan of hot water — better than my boarding school version!

Hollandaise Sauce

Serves 4

Ingredients

	Metric	Imperial	American
large fresh egg yolks	2	2	2
lemon juice	*1 tsp*	*1 tsp*	*1 tsp*
melted butter	*1 tbsp*	*1 tbsp*	*1 tbsp*
seasoning to taste			
softened butter	*75 g*	*3 oz*	*6 tbsp*

Method

Put the yolks, lemon juice, seasoning and melted butter in a bowl standing in a saucepan of hot water. Using a balloon or electric whisk, mix the ingredients and keep whisking while adding the softened butter, a teaspoon at a time. It's very tedious but worth the effort (don't try and hurry the job or the lot will curdle). When the sauce is pale in colour and thick, like mayonnaise, serve immediately. Serve with hot salmon or any poached or baked fish.

Aïoli

This devastatingly fattening, delicious, creamy mayonnaise complements any cold fish or shellfish. It is floated on top of a fish soup — but you must be madly in love with garlic.

Blend 6 crushed cloves of garlic with lemon juice, a pinch of sea salt and one large egg yolk. Using exactly the same method as for mayonnaise, add 300 ml (½ pint/1¼ cups) good olive oil drip by drip by drop at first, then in a continuous stream until a thick and creamy consistency is achieved.

Fish Soup

Serves 4

A wealth of goodness with no rules and regulations as to correct ingredients. Keep the boney fish away if the children or granny are to indulge — a little of the lobster tails, big prawns and scallops may be added for a dinner party where you need to impress the boss — a meal in itself!

You must have onions and garlic (to your own taste) to start. Peel, chop and sauté them in a little butter, about 25 g(1 oz/2 tbsp), and then as a guide add:

Ingredients

	Metric	Imperial	American
prepared mixed fish and shellfish to include cod, whiting, haddock, hake — anything goes	700 g	1½ lb	1½ lb
pinch of saffron			
glass of dry white wine	1	1	1
tomatoes, chopped, or use a tin of peeled tomatoes	2	2	2
tomato purée	2 tbsp	2 tbsp	2 tbsp
fresh herbs if possible, such as tarragon, parsley, dill and a bay leaf			
seasoning to taste			
stock made with vegetable stock cube or Vecon	1 litre	2 pints	5 cups
sea vegetables	25 g	1 oz	1 oz
Aïoli to serve			
a few shrimps or prawns to garnish			

Method

Cut all the fish into bite size pieces, removing any visible bones or skin. If using Conger eel, remember it takes a little longer cooking time than other white fish and should be tossed into the soup pot with the semi cooked onions and garlic, at least 15 minutes before other fish —with stock.

Soak the saffron in the wine for at least 10 minutes before adding to the soup. Put all the fish (not the shellfish), tomato purée and herbs with seasoning into the par-cooked onions and garlic. Add the stock and sea vegetables, bring to the boil, reduce the heat and allow to simmer for 10 minutes before adding the wine and saffron. Cook for a further 5 minutes on simmer, then add any shrimps or prawns or other shellfish to include lobster — if using scallops they take only seconds to cook.

Have 4 large soup bowls warming, coat each dish with a little Aïoli. Spoon the soup into each bowl with care. Garnish and serve immediately with hot crusty bread —no need for butter on your bread.

Note: If you want to make the Aïoli go a little further and reduce the cholesterol, fold into whisked egg whites or a little low-fat natural yogurt.

Chapter 4

A-Z OF OMEGA 3

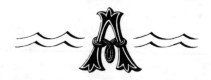

And in the very beginning there must always be shoals of little anchovies!

ANCHOVIES

These tiny, tasty fish are caught in the inshore waters of the North Sea, with the majority very sensibly preferring the warmer waters of the Mediterranean. Because they don't like to travel they are usually found in a tin. If you are lucky enough to find them fresh, just chop off their heads and grill. Serve with a little black pepper and fresh lemon juice. Don't underestimate this little fish — it is packed with OMEGA 3.

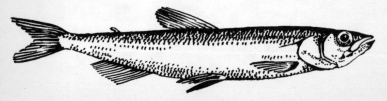

Anchovy

Anchovy and Potato Pie

For everybody too far away from 'anchovy waters', buy two tins and treat the family to this very easy and tasty meal. As fish cooks quickly and potatoes more slowly — make sure the potatoes are sliced very fine.

Serves 3-4

Ingredients

	Metric	Imperial	American
small tins of anchovies, drained	2	2	2
little milk or wine for soaking			
tin of peeled tomatoes, drained	425 g	15 oz	15 oz
fresh tomatoes, skinned	4	4	4
potatoes, peeled and finely sliced	450 g	1 lb	1 lb
cloves of garlic, crushed	2	2	2
a little black pepper			
chopped fresh parsley to garnish			

Method

Soak the anchovies in a little milk or wine for 1 hour. Pour off the liquid which will take away the excess salt. Chop the canned and fresh tomatoes. Grease an ovenproof dish, layer with fish and potatoes, with a sprinkling of garlic and pepper. Top with the tomatoes. Bake in the oven at 200°C (400°F) Gas 6 for 35 minutes. Garnish with chopped parsley and serve.

Arbroath Smokie

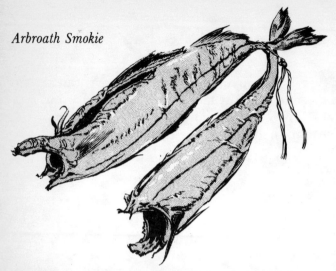

ANGLER FISH   see Monkfish

ARBROATH SMOKIES

Scotland is where you will find smokies — 'hot smoked' small haddock. The fish are beheaded, cleaned and left in dry salt for 1 hour before being tied in pairs and hung over hot smoke. The result produces a mildly smoked fish that can be devoured hot or cold. Due to this method of smoking, it is as well to eat smokies within 48 hours of purchase.

Smokie and Hot Potato

Remove skin and brush the fish lightly with butter. Grill for a few minutes on each side to heat through — remember it has already been cooked over the hot smoke. Serve with a baked jacket potato heaped with a spoonful of fromage frais. A little seasoning and lemon juice don't go amiss.

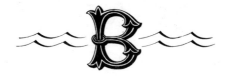

BASS　see Sea Bass

BLACKJACK　see Coley

BLOATER
(Mild Cured Smoked Herring)

omega 3

A fresh herring that has been smoked over oak logs with its innards left inside for extra flavour. Quite popular around East Anglia and most definitely on the breakfast table in the East End of London. My fishmonger friends tell me that a bloater should only be grilled. Open up the fish, remove the innards (you can remove the head if it makes you feel happier), rub both sides of the fish with butter and grill each side for about 3-4 minutes — don't overcook!

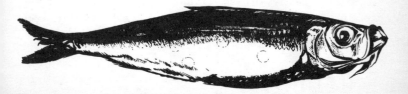

Bloater

Bloater Paste

Stand a bloater in a jug of boiling water for 10 minutes. Remove skin, bones and innards, retrieving all the flesh. Purée the fish with a little pepper and a squeeze of fresh lemon to make it extra tasty. Spread on wholemeal toast or in brown bread sandwiches.

BREAM/SEA BREAM (Porgie)

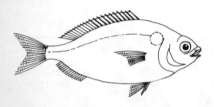

There are many varieties of bream from many parts of the world, but the red one is the best for the table. To be found during the months of June and December in our British waters, the rest of the year they are imported. A fatless fish with an oval body, the best weight is around 400 g (14 oz), they seem to have more flavour than an older fish. They can be cooked whole in foil with a few herbs and trimmings-a-la Français — or are delicious on the barbecue. Whatever way you choose to cook bream, remove the scales. Freshwater bream are quite plentiful in our rivers and streams, with a record weight of 7 kg (about 16 lb) reported. But my friendly angler tells me that when he has caught his whopper, he always throws it back. Is this all to do with the etiquette of angling? I think I would wash my muddy fish very well and get it in the oven!

Grilled Bream

Wash well and, with the innards removed, stuff the belly

of each fish with fresh herbs including tarragon, dill, chervil or just parsley if available. Top with butter (as it is a dry fish), grill each side and serve with fresh lemon and pepper.

BRILL

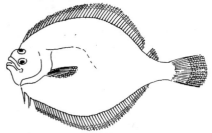

In the main, brill comes from the West Country. A flat fish with a browny top and creamy white underside, it is excellent grilled with a little butter, but it will be necessary to fillet if somebody surprises you with a three pounder or more. Ask your fishmonger to cut the fillets — his knife is better than yours — but don't let him keep the head and bones, they make wonderful gelatinous stock for the base of a good fish sauce.

Steamed Brill Fillets with Apple Mayonnaise

Serves 4

Ingredients

	Metric	Imperial	American
fillets of brill taken from one large fish	4	4	4
fresh lemon juice			
a little black pepper			

a little fresh watercress, samphire or parsley to garnish			
Sauce:			
stewed Bramley apples, unsweetened, still warm	225 g	8 oz	1 cup
Wobbly mayonnaise (see page 16)	2 tbsp	2 tbsp	2 tbsp
Dijon mustard	1 tsp	1 tsp	1 tsp
pinch cayenne pepper			

Method

Rub each fillet with lemon juice and sprinkle with black pepper, steam for 4-5 minutes — don't overcook. Purée all the sauce ingredients. Put the fillets on individual plates with the garnish. Serve the sauce in a separate bowl.

BROWN SHRIMPS   see Shrimps

BUCKLING

A herring left whole with it's innards intact (all to give a more meaty flavour), salted slightly before hot smoking over wood chippings. To serve, remove the innards and serve with horseradish sauce and brown bread. Plenty of OMEGA 3.

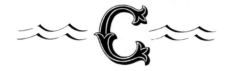

CARP

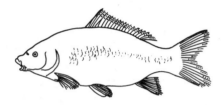

Oily freshwater fish that is caught in rivers
and lakes. Monks were farming carp in the
ponds of monasteries many moons ago.
Apart from pike and salmon, carp is the largest fish in the
British Isles, weighing anything from 4.5 kg (10 lb) to over
18 kg (40 lb). It makes an excellent fish for a party, cooked
and served whole. All the scales must be removed before
any method of cooking.

Boiled Carp (Karpion Mevushal)

Serves 6

Ingredients

	Metric	Imperial	American
freshly caught carp, descaled	2 kg	4 lb	4 lb
coarse sea salt	2 tbsp	2 tbsp	2 tbsp
large onions, peeled and thinly sliced	2	2	2

carrots, peeled and finely slivered	5	5	5
celeriac root, peeled and finely sliced	1	1	1
parsnips, peeled and finely sliced	2	2	2
tomatoes, halved	5	5	5
pepper to taste with 1 tablespoon sugar			

Method

Cover the fish with salt and leave to stand for 1 hour, then refresh under cold water. Place the vegetables in a fish kettle and lay the fish on top. Place the tomatoes on top of the fish with a little pepper and sugar. Cover with water and cook for 50 minutes, covered. Lift out the fish with loving care and give the vegetables a little extra cooking time if necessary.

A little watercress, mustard and cress or parsley can be used as a garnish with wedges of lemon. Plenty of OMEGA 3.

CATFISH (Wolf Fish)

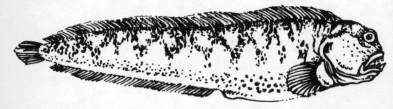

In the days of yore, this ugly brute (really quite delicious to eat) was commonly known as dogfish or rock salmon. Worldwide today, the term catfish usually refers to a fresh-water fish that is flown in from as far afield as America, mostly as frozen steaks or fillets. A deep sea species is found off the coast of Greenland and it is now packed into very convenient packs for the freezer cabinets — but called a rockfish. But just to add a little confusion to your life, if you are passing through Yorkshire, you will always be able to find wolf fish; prepared into fillets so as not to frighten the kiddies. It's a good fish to buy for the children and the elderly because it is packed with fine protein and has only one centre 'bone' that isn't even a real bone but cartilage. No, not Wolf Pie — Woof Pie.

Woof Pie from Yorkshire

Serves 4

Ingredients

	Metric	Imperial	American
a knob of butter			
catfish fillets, dredged in flour	450 g	1 lb	1 lb
hard boiled eggs, sliced	2	2	2
large leek, blanched part only, finely chopped	1	1	1
milk, skimmed can be used	200 ml	7 fl oz	⅞ cup
seasoning to taste			
home made or ready made short crust pastry	225 g	8 oz	½ lb

Method

Butter a pie dish well, layer the fish with the eggs and leek. Pour in the milk, add seasoning and remainder of butter. Roll out the pastry to make a pie crust with two holes for steam to escape (or use a pie funnel). Bake in the oven at 190°C (375°F) Gas 5 for 45-50 minutes. Serve hot or cold.

CHICKEN TURBOT   see Turbot

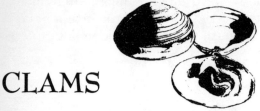

CLAMS

They are sold live, but are easy to cook by popping into boiling water for a couple of minutes until the shells are open. Really tasty with a dash of vinegar — or enjoy them raw like an oyster with a squeeze of fresh lemon. Examine clams before cooking and make sure you discard any with a broken shell and those that do not close back tightly when the shell is tapped. It's a good idea to soak them for an hour in clean salt water to allow the live clams to spit out any sand. Excellent in a fish soup or stew. The extra large American very hard shelled type are a must for chowder.

Clams with Pasta Shells

Serves 4

Ingredients

	Metric	Imperial	American
medium onions, peeled and finely chopped	2	2	2
cloves of garlic, chopped into small pieces	4	4	4
cold pressed virgin olive oil (wonderful flavour and aroma)	2 tbsp	2 tbsp	2 tbsp

tomatoes, skinned and chopped, or tinned	*450 g*	*1 lb*	*1 lb*
black pepper			
fresh clams	*700 g*	*1 ½ lb*	*1 ½ lb*
pasta shells or twirls	*550 g*	*1 ¼ lb*	*1 ¼ lb*
chopped fresh basil, if available			

Method

Fry the onions and garlic in oil over gentle heat for about 5 minutes. Add the tomatoes and pepper, cover and simmer for 20 minutes. Cook the clams and drain, see left, reserving about 7-8 tablespoons of the water to add to the tomatoes. Cook the pasta as directed, drain well. To serve, just mix everything together, including the basil, and enjoy.

COALFISH   (**Pollock**)   see Coley

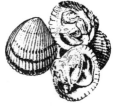

COCKLES

'a-r cocos yn byrlymu ytywod' thought Dylan Thomas, as he wrote 'Under Milkwood'. Molluscs can be found in abundance along the Gower coastline and on many other sandy shores in Britain. Try a fry-up of cockles and laverbread. Toss cockles into fresh pasta and give your guests the time of their lives with a tooth pick.

Freshly boiled they are quite delicious with just a little shake of vinegar and seasoning. To get rid of the sand, soak overnight in clean water with salt.A rich source of iron and selenium; you can afford to eat plenty.

Cockles & Eggs (Cocos ac Wyau)

Serves 4

Ingredients

	Metric	Imperial	American
cockles, uncooked	2.4 litres	4 pts	4 pts
eggs, whisked well	4	4	4
black pepper			
to taste			
butter	25 g	1 oz	2 tbsp

Method

Cover the cockles with water, give a good shake of the pan and then pour off water and replace with fresh. Bring water to the boil and cook cockles for two further minutes only. (Don't overcook to make them tough.)

Pick cockles from shells whilst warm — Granny will love this job with the children. — Place cockles in colender and wash well once again in warm water to remove any remaining sand. Drain well and pat dry with kitchen paper. In a teflon coated frying pan, heat cockles through in the butter and pour over the eggs.

When the eggs have set, add a few turns of the black pepper mill and serve with Laver Bread (Bara Lawr).

COD

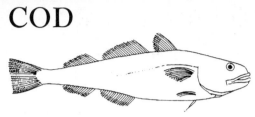

Quality fish with firm white flesh and not to be messed about with in pies, pizza and stew. The finest fried cod with chips (grilled if you prefer) can be found in London at Seafresh, Wilton Road. I know why the cod is so damned good — because it is caught in Scotland on the Monday and is on the table by Tuesday — you can't have anything fresher than that!

On the days you don't eat fish, take cod liver oil in liquid or capsule form for your daily dose of OMEGA 3. (OMEGA 3 is nothing new, Granny has been taking it from the bottle for years.)

Simple Cod Bake with Mushrooms

Serves 2

Ingredients

	Metric	Imperial	American
really fresh cod fillet, skin removed	450 g	1 lb	1 lb
seasoning to taste			
medium onion, peeled and finely chopped	1	1	1
button mushrooms, wiped and sliced	100 g	4 oz	1 cup
butter	50 g	2 oz	¼ cup
flour	25 g	1 oz	¼ cup
skimmed milk	300 ml	½ pint	1¼ cups
chopped fresh parsley			

Method

Place the fish on foil and season well. Fry the onion and mushrooms in half the butter for 4 minutes, then lift on to the fish. Seal up the foil. Bake in the oven at 190°C (375°F) Gas 5 for 20 minutes.

Add the remaining butter to the frying pan, blend in the flour, and give the pan a whirl round. Gradually add the milk and plenty of parsley to make a smooth sauce. When the fish is cooked, make a hole in the foil and allow any juices to run into the sauce. Give the sauce a good stir and serve with the fish. If serving with mashed potatoes, don't bother to add butter and milk to the potatoes — the rich sauce will trickle through on the plate to give that extra flavour.

COD, SALT

Preserving fish in salt has been known through the ages. Some supermarkets can supply, but it is more popular in Chinese supermarkets. I always see plenty in Spain where it is very popular.

Soak salt cod well for 24 hours at least — 48 to be on the safe side — keep changing the cold water.

To cook: cover with fresh water, bring to the boil, then remove from the heat and allow to cool. Flake the fish, removing the skin or bones.

Salt Cod with Tomatoes

Pop cooked salt cod into a frying pan with a little olive oil and toss gently for 1 minute over a low heat. Add a tin of chopped tomatoes, a little chopped parsley, seasoning to taste and a glass of sherry. The total cooking time is only 6 minutes. Serve with noodles or pasta shells.

COD'S ROE

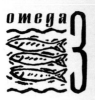

'Poor man's caviare' in the North when served in slices with a dash of vinegar, salt and pepper — plus the Hovis of course!

Cod Roe Fritters

Makes 4 fritters

Ingredients

	Metric	Imperial	American
boiled cod's roe, sliced into 4 pieces	275 g	10 oz	10 oz
a little groundnut oil for frying			
Batter:			
flour	50 g	2 oz	½ cup
large egg	1	1	1

Method

For the batter, blend the flour with the egg. Add sufficient cold water to make a batter of coating consistency. Allow to stand for at least 50 minutes.

Heat the oil until it is about to smoke. Dip the roe pieces in the batter and shallow fry both sides for about 4 minutes. Lift on to kitchen paper to drain for 3 seconds. Serve immediately with wedges of lemon or brown sauce.

COD'S ROE, SMOKED

Smoked cod's roe is expensive. Slice smoked roe very thinly for a special starter, and serve with lambs' lettuce and watercress, slices of lemon and freshly ground black pepper. It is also the basic ingredient for that famous Greek dip Taramasalata.

COLEY (Coalfish)

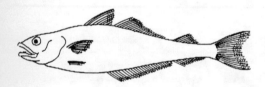

If this fish was expensive, more would be sold. But because of the combination of cheap price and mucky colour, people are very wary. A member of the cod family, also called saithe, coalfish and blackjack; rest assured, the colour changes to white on cooking and the flavour is excellent. Ideal for pies, pizza, stews and soup. A good fish that is full of protein and no fat.

Cheap and Cheerful Fish Pie

Serves 6

Ingredients

	Metric	Imperial	American
coley, skin removed	*700 g*	*1½ lb*	*1½ lb*
bay leaves	*2*	*2*	*2*

skimmed milk	450 ml	¾ pint	2 cups
seasoning to taste			
dried seaweed (sea vegetables)	50 g	2 oz	2 oz
hard-boiled eggs, coarsely chopped	2	2	2
leeks, blanched part, thinly sliced	2	2	2
butter	25 g	1 oz	2 tbsp
flour	25 g	1 oz	¼ cup
parsley, finely chopped	25 g	1 oz	1 oz
grated nutmeg to taste			
boiled potatoes, mashed	800 g	1¾ lb	1¾ lb
tomatoes	2	2	2

Method

Wash the fish in cold water, then cook with the bay leaves, half the milk and seasoning for about 7 minutes. Lift the fish from the stock, remove any skin and bones, then flake.

Put the seaweed into cold water to soak for 5 minutes while cooking the fish. Drain and cut into small pieces with scissors, then mix into the fish with the eggs. Sauté the leeks in the butter for 5 minutes over a gentle heat. Shake in the flour and, stirring continuously, mix in the milk reserved from the cooked fish with remaining milk. Stir to make a smooth leek sauce. Mix in the parsley, adjust the seasoning, add the nutmeg and remove the bay leaves.

To assemble the pie, mix the fish into the sauce and pour into a pie dish. Top with potatoes. Halve the tomatoes and arrange on top of the potatoes. Sprinkle with cheese. Bake in the oven at 200°C (400°F) Gas 6 for 20-25 minutes until the top sizzles into the potatoes.

CONGER EEL

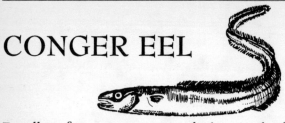

Excellent for stews, soups and pies. As the flesh is a little coarse, always ask for the middle steaks — they are less bony than the tail end. I maintain that the only fish that needs cooking well is conger eel, opposed to any other fish or shellfish. A microwave does not overcook conger eel as it can do with other fish.

Microwave Conger Casserole

Serves 4

Ingredients

	Metric	Imperial	American
medium onions, peeled and sliced	2	2	2
cloves of garlic, chopped	4	4	4
a little corn oil or butter to sauté			
steaks of conger eel, 175g(6oz/6oz) each	4	4	4
sticks of celery, chopped	4	4	4
large carrots, peeled and sliced to match celery	2	2	2
fresh parsley, chopped	25 g	1 oz	1 oz
medium parsnip, peeled and cut into cubes to match carrots	1	1	1
seasoning to taste			
dry cider	300 ml	½ pint	1¼ cups
tomato purée (optional)	1 tbsp	1 tbsp	1 tbsp

Method

Sauté the onions and garlic in the oil or butter for 4 minutes. Place the conger steaks in the pan and brown each side for 2 minutes. Turn ingredients into a microwaveproof casserole and add the remainder of the ingredients. Cook on High for 15 minutes. A few thin slices of potato can be placed in the casserole if there is room.

CRAB

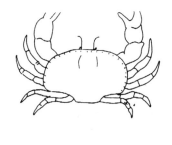

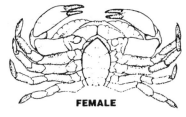

FEMALE

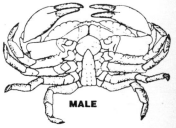

MALE

A crustacean! There are three main kinds of crab to be found around our British waters and the most popular must be the common brown crab — the one that becomes more red in colour when cooked.

Did you know that a crab changes it's shell every year? And did you know, at the end of twelve month period, it will begin to form a new shell inside the old? When the new shell is completely formed, the old shell is shed; the crab crawls under the rocks, fills the new shell with water, inflating it to a size the crab will itself fill. Would you believe that within two or three days this soft shell will harden like a rock — but this is not the time to buy your crab for the table — nothing in the shell but water! The best time to buy a crab is around spring time, just before the old shell falls because it is just so packed full of delicious meat.

So how do you know which is the right crab so packed with meat? Look for a tough shell with a few barnacles. Avoid light, milky coloured shells! Lift your crab and if it feels much heavier than the given weight it will be packed with meat. Give a little shake; you will hear water in a crab with a new shell! Turn the crab over; if the join where the shell starts is slightly open it means the crab is bursting at the seams with delicious meat — pay for it quick and get it home for tea!

There are two kinds of meat in a crab; white claw meat and the brown meat in the body shell. A cock crab has the large claws with plenty of white meat as opposed to a hen crab who has less white meat and more brown in the shell. You can tell a cock crab by the small flap on the underside — the hen has a much larger, broad flap (see illustrations).

Your friendly fishmonger will always boil and dress your fresh crab. However, to dress a crab yourself, prise the top shell from the body to which the claws and little legs are attached. Immediately remove the gills, recognizable by their greyish colour — NOT nice to eat! We don't talk 'dead man's fingers' any more — puts people off! But every other scrap of flesh, be it brown or white, and not shell, you can eat — promise. (The Japanese eat the lot!)

Scrape out all the dark meat, set aside. Clean out the meat from the centre of the body, mix with the meat from top shell. Twist the claws and legs from the body, crack with nutcrackers to enable all the white meat to be extracted with ease. Cut the cartilage between the pincers, open the pincers and the meat should come away with great ease in one piece — don't forget there is succulent meat where the legs were attached. Don't buy one crab for four servings; a 1 kg (2 lb) crab should yield about 325 g (11-12 oz) of meat —only enough for two.

Crab Tea for Two

Ingredients

	Metric	Imperial	American
slices Spanish onion, finely chopped, or 2 spring onions, chopped	2	2	2
finely chopped fresh parsley	2 tbsp	2 tbsp	2 tbsp
juice of lemon	½	½	½
Worcestershire sauce (optional)	4 drops	4 drops	4 drops
large prepared crab, white and brown meat separated	1	1	1
fresh brown breadcrumbs	2 tbsp	2 tbsp	2 tbsp
Wobbly mayonnaise (see page 16)	1½ tbsp	1½ tbsp	1½ tbsp
vinegar	2 tbsp	2 tbsp	2 tbsp
a little seasoning			

Method

Mix the onion, most of the parsley, the lemon juice and Worcestershire sauce into the white meat. Fold the breadcrumbs into the mayonnaise with vinegar and seasoning, then fold into the brown meat. Wash the shell and dry. Arrange the brown meat in the middle of the shell, surround with the white meat. Garnish with the reserved parsley. Serve with a salad.

CRAB, CROMER

Buy two of these cooked little gems and give yourself a treat. And so easy to prepare yourself. If you prise the top shell from the bottom you will see the little soft grey feathery gills that lie each side of the body, gently push these away and discard — you can eat the rest. Push out as much meat as you can and mix with a little vinegar, pepper and salt.

CRAB, SPIDER

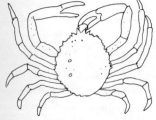

Delicious to eat, but very fiddly — that is why we lazy British don't bother with them. Most of the catch comes from Cornwall and is packed off alive to the Continent where they don't mind the fiddle. A small beach crab can also be used for this recipe.

Spider Crab Soup

Serves 4

Ingredients

	Metric	Imperial	American
large onion, peeled and chopped	1	1	1
cloves of garlic, chopped	4	4	4
cold pressed virgin olive oil	2 tbsp	2 tbsp	2 tbsp

sticks celery, chopped	2	2	2
carrot, peeled and chopped	1	1	1
water	900 ml	1½ pints	3¾ cups
spider crab	1	1	1
glass dry white wine	1	1	1
black pepper to taste			
single cream	100 ml	3½ fl oz	7 tbsp

Method

Sauté the onion and garlic in the oil for 4 minutes over a gentle heat. Add the celery and carrot, cook for 5 minutes before adding the water. Cover and allow to simmer for 20 minutes. Break the shell of the crab into at least 4 pieces and add to the pan with the separated legs. Bring to the boil and take off the heat immediately. Turn all the ingredients into a blender or food processor, (this may have to be done in 3 batches), then run the machine to break down the crab with shells. Turn these ingredients into a large sieve and press down well to extract all the goodness and flavours. Return the precious juices and flavours to a saucepan, stir in the wine and bring slowly to the boil. Adjust seasoning at this stage, stir in the cream — don't boil — and serve in 4 warmed soup bowls.

CRAB, VELVET

Available from October to June. If you happen to be in the Orkney Isles, a self imposed ban operates during the summer months. However, there are plenty more on the west coast of Scotland. But do we indulge? No! This delicate, delicious crab gets packed live on a Tuesday to arrive in Spain on Thursday — and the Spanish want more, olé!

CRAWFISH (Spring Lobster)

Often mistaken for lobster, although it is a bit 'all body and large front claws'. For the lazy lobster eater, this fat crustacean is the answer. All the meat is in the body and saves nutcrackers and fiddly picking to get the last bits out of the claws. No fat, lots of protein and a great shellfish to look out for, especially when on hols in Cornwall.

Crawfish Au Natural For Two

If you can't cope with cooking a live crawfish, order one from your friendly fishmonger and he will cook it. When you call to collect, get him to cut straight through the middle of the shell — unless you are a chef. Take the crawfish home, heat, extract the meat and slice. Line 2 plates with shredded raddiccio, chicory, lollo rosso (different pretty lettuce to make everything more romantic). Arrange the meat on the lettuce and add wedges of lemon. Serve with home made Wobbly mayonnaise (see page 16) and a bottle of Canard-Duchêne — well chilled!

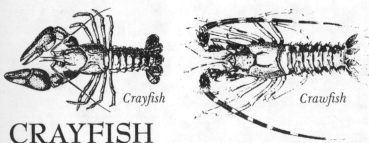

Crayfish   *Crawfish*

CRAYFISH

Try to catch a few of these freshwater crustaceans before they are packed off live to the Continent where those foreigners know what makes for a gourmandise delight. In

1980, the British Crayfish Marketing Association was formed to allow the housewife to get a 'look in'. You can usually find crayfish in season at a really classy fish restaurant where the chef should know how to serve them to their best advantage — and that is not in a stew! Buy your crayfish live for the best flavour. Cook just before serving by plunging into boiling water (court-bouillon if preferred). Boil for 2-3 minutes, depending on size. Never overcook as the meat will go chewy — slightly undercooking encourages a more succulent texture. Twist off the tails, remove shells, then pull out the dark thread-like veins. Arrange on a bed of various shredded lettuce and serve immediately with fresh lemon mayonnaise (see page 17).

Crayfish the Scandinavian Way

Assemble a huge pile of crayfish cooked in salty water and beer. Serve with brown bread and butter, a good sprinkle of chopped fresh dill and wedges of lemon.

CUTTLEFISH

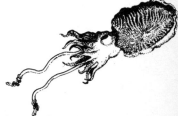

Cook as for Squid. They both need to be cooked very quickly or for a long time; for some reason I am unable to fathom out, any cooking time in between make them very tough. Don't be put off by the untidy tentacles and fat body, if you can't find a fishmonger to prepare it for you, there are plenty of prepared frozen in the supermarket. You can stuff a cuttlefish with chopped fish and herbs — quite delicious. The ink makes a fine sauce when cooked with onions, wine and cream, so don't take fright and throw it down the sink.

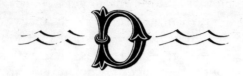

DAB

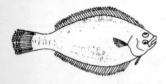

Lots of little dabs for a quid (£); a sign so often seen along the Kent coastline. A very underestimated little flat fish with a delicate flavour and not to be ignored — especially at a few pence a fish! Cook whole; too small to bother with fillets.

Fried Dabs for Breakfast

Ingredients

	Metric	Imperial	American
dabs per person	2	2	2
seasoned flour			
groundnut oil or a little butter for frying			

Method

Remove the heads from the fish and descale the rough side. Wash away the innards under cold running water, then pat dry with kitchen paper. Dredge with seasoned flour. Heat oil or butter in a frying pan and, when just beginning to smoke, fry both sides of the fish for about 4 minutes. Serve immediately with tomato sauce or lemon, hunks of new bread or toast.

Note: Fried fish is tasty, but cook quickly each side at the correct temperature (just when the fat begins to smoke), this way a seal is made to prevent fish taking a drenching. To leave fish bubbling for 15 minutes spells a horror story — especially for the waistline.

DOGFISH   see Huss — plenty of OMEGA 3.

DORY   see John Dory

DOVER SOLE

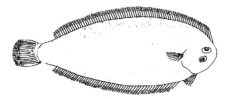

Acknowledged to be the best from the sole family. Called Dover sole because Dover was once the most efficient outlet to get this species of fish to London. The sole is a prize fish from any British waters, but the best come from Torbay in Devon; and you won't see many of this kind on the fishmonger's slab in the Midlands. A Torbay sole is assured to be plump with a tasty flesh to the edge of every fin — and the French have the pick of the shoal. Our friends across the Channel know the best and they are prepared to pay the price for the best. The only way I know to cook a sole is to

grill. No dressing! No sauce! No fancy camouflage —
nothing – just fresh lemon.

Grilled Sole

One sole per person — at least 2 days old; if you try
cleaning a sole the day it is caught it will slip straight
down the plug-hole. The flavour improves by keeping it
a couple of days from being caught — NOT from when
you get it home from your fishmonger.

Remove the dark skin, your fishmonger will do this
for you, but keep the white skin because it helps to keep
the fish in shape and adds flavour, you can grill skinned
fillets but the taste is not so good. Brush the fish with
softened butter, pop under a hot grill and cook both
sides for 4-5 minutes (depending on size). Serve
immediately with wedges of lemon and a green side
salad.

DUBLIN BAY PRAWNS
(Norway Lobster)

Better known as 'scampi'. The word scampi (to mean the
whole tail) is Italian; the French call them langoustine, if
you are puzzled on a day trip to Calais — and the French
love their langoustines. Just to confuse the whole issue, the
correct scientific name is Nephrops (norvegicus) or Norway
lobster.

Although this wonderful shellfish is landed in other
countries, including Spain and Italy, landings in Europe
are dominated by those from Scotland; with a fair catch
from around the waters of North East England and
Northern Ireland — so why don't we see Nephrops alive
'en masse' on our fishmonger's slab?

In this country, only the tails of this crustacea are used;

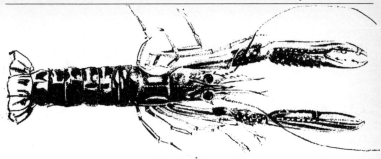

Dublin Bay Prawn

and there are plenty of frozen supplies in the supermarket. If you keep your eyes peeled, you can find a few live Nephrops — recognizable by their pink fat bodies with long red claws — and they still remain pink when cooked for a minute in boiling water.

Fantastically delicious lightly brushed with oil and grilled whole over a barbecue on skewers — especially when served with chilled Prosper Maufoux Bourgogne (Chardonnay).

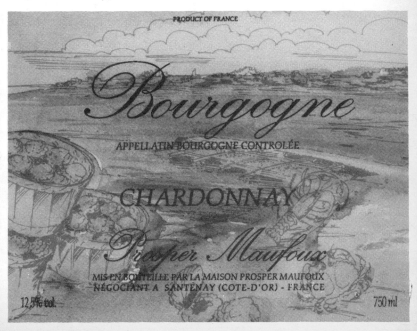

Scampi in a Basket

Serves 2

Ingredients

	Metric	Imperial	American
Dublin Bay prawns	*16*	*16*	*16*
oil for deep frying			
Batter:			
olive oil or a good vegetable oil	*1 tbsp*	*1 tbsp*	*1 tbsp*
cold water	*4 tbsp*	*4 tbsp*	*4 tbsp*
plain flour	*50 g*	*2 oz*	*½ cup*
pinch of salt and shake of black pepper			
egg white	*1*	*1*	*1*

Method

Blend the oil and water into the flour with seasoning and allow to stand for at least 50 minutes. Whisk the egg white until stiff and fold into the batter just before frying.

Have a deep fryer at the ready with oil at the right temperature for deep frying — about 180-198°C (350-390°F); the oil will let off just a hint of smoke but it should not be bubbling. Deep frying this way seals the batter without allowing the oil to penetrate into the fish — all to make for healthier eating. Dip the prawns into the batter and fry for about 3-4 minutes. When the prawns are cooked, lift with a slotted spoon on to kitchen paper to remove excess oil. Serve immediately. Please do not keep warm, re-heat or serve cold — Ruination! Serve immediately with wedges of lemon and brown bread and butter.

EELS

A true cockney delicacy — freshly killed and cooked while you wait. The Belgians prize our live eels, they make their special pie and use them to liven up a fish stew. We are now getting the eels back into pies —removing the steak and kidney. Eels are reputed to be the most nutritious of all fish!

Jellied Eels

Don't be put off by the fact that you must kill your eels just seconds before they go into the cooking pot; your friendly fishmonger will perform the last rites, including chopping them into manageable pieces. Don't let him remove the skin before chopping. This is the cockney secret of that delicious and nutritious jelly. Run straight home, get the pot on the stove with chopped onion, herbs, seasoning and sufficient water to cover the eel and simmer for 35 minutes. When the eel is tender, lift into little pots, leave the stock to boil rapidly uncovered for 1 minute, to reduce a little, then pour over the eel. Serve when the jelly has set.

Slimming with Eels

They are low in fat and high in nutritional value.

Serves 2

Ingredients

	Metric	Imperial	American
large onion, peeled and sliced	1	1	1
carrots, peeled and sliced	2	2	2
medium leeks, blanched part only, sliced	2	2	2
butter	25 g	1 oz	2 tbsp
eel, cut into manageable pieces	450 g	1 lb	1 lb
bottle red wine (alcohol reduces calories when reaching a certain temperature in cooking)	½	½	½
chopped parsley, bay leaf fresh or dried thyme			
seasoning to taste			
a drop of brandy (optional)			

Method

Mix the onion, carrots and leeks together and gently fry in the butter. Lay the eel on top of the vegetables and cook each side for about 4 minutes. Pour in the wine, add the herbs and seasoning to taste. Cover and simmer on top of the cooker, or pop in the oven and cook for 45 minutes. Remove the lid and add that dash of brandy, cook for a further 3-4 minutes. Serve with mashed potatoes — or forget the potatoes and have an extra steak of eel, more protein, fewer calories.

ELVERS

Elvers are baby eels that are caught in rivers when returning from the seas to their parents' old habitat. Our British elvers are also found in great quantity on the dining table of the French, Spanish and Belgian gourmets. We don't eat elvers in this country — because we don't know what to do with them; nobody ever tells us how to cook them. They are simply delicious when dredged in seasoned flour, deep fried and served as a starter.

Watch out for the Severn poachers as they hustle their night catch through that Channel Tunnel to the markets on the other side — they'll earn themselves a pile of ecus!

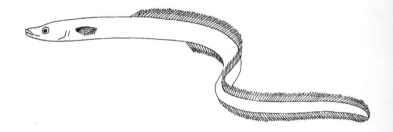

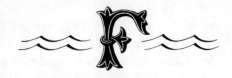

FINNAN HADDOCK

Beware of brightly dyed haddock — a completely different 'kettle of fish' to the real thing. In the past when there was an abundance of fish to be found around our coastal waters, salting and smoking were a very excellent means of preservation. Finnan haddock (Finny haddie) is beheaded, split down the middle with the backbone left to the right side and the tails kept on. Left in a smoke hole for days, the peat or wood ash smokes the haddock making it quite unnecessary for lengthy cooking time when preparing for that very traditional breakfast. A good source of OMEGA 3.

Finnan Haddock for Breakfast

Ingredients

	Metric	Imperial	American
whole fish per person	*1*	*1*	*1*
skimmed milk for poaching			
a shake of white pepper			
small pats of butter	*2*	*2*	*2*

Method

Place the fish in sufficient milk to almost cover. Add the

pepper and butter. Bring the milk to the boil, reduce heat and simmer until cooked (really meaning until well warmed through). Don't overcook, minutes only should heat a medium size haddock.

Note: I only like a microwave oven when the word steaming or boiling comes into a fish recipe. For many pieces of fish or shellfish a microwave is all to quick and will overcook the fish. Cook Finnan haddock in a microwave on High for 2-3 minutes, depending on size. Allow to stand for 2 minutes before removing the skin.

Cullen Skink

Here is Joseph Robertson's famous recipe.

Serves 4

Ingredients

	Metric	Imperial	American
smoked haddock (Finnan on the bone preferred)	*1*	*1*	*1*
potatoes	*450 g*	*1 lb*	*1 lb*
medium onion, peeled and chopped	*1*	*1*	*1*
butter	*25-50 g*	*1-2 oz*	*2-4 tbsp*
milk	*600ml*	*1 pint*	*2½ cups*
seasoning to taste			

Method

Skin the haddock, then place in a pan with water to cover. Bring to boil and cook for 5-10 minutes until ready. Take the fish from the pan and remove the bones. Return the bones to the pan and boil for 45-50 minutes.

Meanwhile, boil and strain the potatoes and onion. Mash well, adding some of the butter. Flake the fish. Strain the bone stock, add the warmed milk, then the fish. Stir in the hot mashed potatoes to give a creamy thickness. Stir in the last of the butter. Add seasoning to taste. Serve hot with brown crusty rolls.

FLAKE   see Huss — both a source of **OMEGA** 3.

FLOUNDER

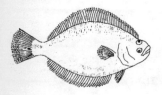

Also called flukes by the folks from Flookburgh. A flat fish and the poor relation from the flat fish family. I would always prize my happy smiling fish, found with my melange of dab, plaice and herring, sold to me from the back of a van in the Dungeness area of Kent. When making my first enquiries as to how to cook flounder, I was always told not to bother due to the tastelessness flavour compared to a plaice. If you are lucky enough to catch a flounder, first give it a good wash under the cold water tap. Trim the fins, rub with butter and cook under or on a grill. Serve with plenty of fresh lemon. You could fry the fillets of a large fish in corn oil, first skinned and coated in fine breadcrumbs.

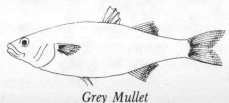

Grey Mullet

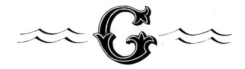

GARFISH

A member of the eel family and very bony.
Cook as Eel. Plenty of OMEGA 3 so well
worth eating.

GRAYLING   see Trout

GREY MULLET

Most surely a fish to be cooked whole. Plenty
can be found around the South and East
coasts. Needs washing very well as this fish
enjoys life in thick mud. Authentic Taramasalata is made
with the roe of grey mullet. Ask you fishmonger to clean
your fish — I don't go for the idea of cooking this fish with
the innards intact, even though they are supposed to make
for a better flavour.

What ever way you cook the fish, remove the scales
before you start, and trim the fins. Rub with lemon and
marjoram and cook on the barbecue; no fat or oil is needed.
This is an oily fish that has plenty of OMEGA 3 — just what
the Family Heart Association ordered.

Baked Grey Mullet

Ingredients

	Metric	Imperial	American
fresh herbs to include parsley, dill and tarragon			
grey mullet per person, cleaned with head intact	1	1	1
lemon slices			
a little white pepper			

Method

Stuff the herbs into the belly of each fish with the lemon, shake the pepper and seal in foil. Bake in the oven at 200°C (400°F) Gas 6 for 15-20 minutes — depending on the size of fish.

Note: The smaller to medium sized fish are reputed to have more flavour than the granny in the shoal.

GURNARD

A very ugly fish, found around Cornwall and Devon, you do get both grey and red gurnard (also called gurnet), and sometimes even a yellow variety. The flesh is quite similar to mullet but it is a bony fish and not really suitable for children. I am told that they are simply delicious if cooked 'au naturel' on the barbecue. No messing with plates or cutlery, just pierce through with a long wooden pick and cook — eat with your fingers. Also easy to bake in the oven.

I am also informed by Peter Davidson from Dengie Shellfish at Burnham-on-Crouch that the big fish were always pounced upon by the old fishing boat skippers to bake whole in the oven — perks of the job.

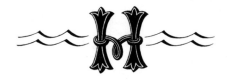

HADDOCK

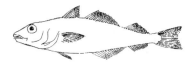

The mighty fish of the North — and 'Fish and Chips'. A round white fish from the cod family with very little fat but plenty of protein. To distinguish it from other members of the family, there is a black stripe running along each side and St Peter once again left his two thumb prints. Haddock loves the deep and cold waters of the Artic — a good reason for him staying away from the Mediterranean.

Steaks or fillets of fish can be boiled, grilled, baked, stewed or made into a pile of goujons; but Haddock and Chips must have been the very beginning of one of our great British institutions.

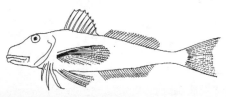

Gurnard

Fish and Chips

Serves 4

Ingredients

	Metric	Imperial	American
thick fillets of haddock, skin removed	4	4	4
Batter:			
plain flour	100 g	4 oz	1 cup
half beer and half water	150 ml	¼ pint	⅔ cup
a little seasoned flour			
groundnut oil for frying			

Method

To make the batter, mix all the ingredients well and allow to stand for at least 30 minutes before use. Wash the fillets under the cold tap, then pat dry.

The secret of perfect batter, which stays crisp on the outside but does not penetrate the fish with oil, is to get the oil at the right temperature, about 180-189°C (350-390°F); the oil will just gently start to smoke when ready. Dip the prepared fish into the batter and lower into the pan to cook, turning during the cooking time if necessary. Depending on the size of the fillets, cooking time should be about 6-7 minutes. You can tell when the fish is cooked because the batter will have risen and be crisp and golden. Don't leave the cooked fish hanging around — straight from the pan to the table, otherwise the batter will become soggy. Serve with chips.

HADDOCK, SMOKED
see also Finnan Haddock

Look out for 'real' smoked haddock, and today it is not easy to find. In days of yore it was popular for the fishmonger to have his own smoke hole where he smoked his own fish over peat, oak dust or wood chippings for his smokies or buckling. The flavour of 'real' smoked fish as opposed to the dyed yellow fish is magnificent; nothing to compare.

The North — that is above Watford Gap, Chertsey in Surrey, and Herne Bay and Flimwell in Kent — with nothing in between, still sport a few good fishmongers with a smoke hole to supply smoked fish.

Smoked Haddock Soufflé

Serves 4

To make a good smoked haddock soufflé you must use the 'real' smoked haddock.

Ingredients

	Metric	Imperial	American
smoked haddock to give rich smoky flavour	*275 g*	*10 oz*	*10 oz*
milk for poaching	*150 ml*	*¼ pint*	*⅔ cup*
butter	*25 g*	*1 oz*	*2 tbsp*
flour	*25 g*	*1 oz*	*¼ cup*
very fresh eggs, separated	*4*	*4*	*4*
(left out of refrigerator for 1 hour before use)			
Cheddar cheese, grated	*50 g*	*2 oz*	*½ cup*
freshly grated nutmeg to taste			
pinch of salt (sea salt if available)			
black pepper to taste			

Method

A good tip taught to me by a famous Swiss chef is to well butter the soufflé dish and stand it in the freezer for at least 30 minutes before use. Any kind of soufflé will come away when serving 'as clean as a whistle'.

Preheat the oven to 180°C (350°F) Gas 4 before you prepare the soufflé — a vital clue to a good result. Butter an 18 cm (7 inch) soufflé dish.

Poach the fish in the milk for 5 minutes. Lift with a slotted spoon and reserve the milk. Remove any visible bones and skin, then flake the flesh. Melt the butter in a pan and blend in the flour over a gentle heat until smooth. Gradually stir in the reserved milk to make a smooth sauce. Beat the egg yolks, add to the sauce with the cheese, nutmeg, salt and pepper, stirring continuously over gentle heat. Cook for 3 minutes, then remove from the heat. Fold in the fish. Whisk the whites until stiff and, with loving care, fold the fish mix into the whites. Pour into the prepared dish. Cook on the middle shelf for 25 minutes. Serve immediately.

HAKE

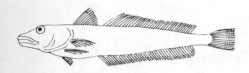

A round member of the cod family, very streamlined in shape due to him not carrying any fat. Certainly a fish that springs up all over the world on the menu; but the hake caught in our own waters both North and South must be a superior quality. Good for invalids when boiled — but very dull! Hake can be used in a pie, soup, curry, quiche, pizza, stew, ceviche, paellas, fried, baked, grilled and poached.

Creamy Hake Bake

Serves 4

Ingredients

	Metric	Imperial	American
softened butter	50 g	2 oz	¼ cup
carton fromage frais, virtually fat free	200 g	7 oz	7 oz
little cornflour or flour			
grated Parmesan cheese	50 g	2 oz	½ cup
seasoning to taste			
hake steaks or fillets	4	4	4

Method

Stir together the butter, fromage frais (mixed with a little cornflour or flour to prevent curdling during cooking) and cheese with the seasoning. Leave the skin on the fish to hold its shape. Place the fish in an ovenproof gratin dish and top with the sauce. Bake in the oven at 180°C (350°F) Gas 4 for 25 minutes.

HALIBUT

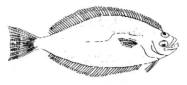

The most vital part of this flat fish must be the liver. Halibut orange oil capsules were freely distributed during the war years to all children and expectant mums — Vitamin C and OMEGA 3. If you can't enjoy fish daily, feed the family with the capsules! Get the fishmonger to cut out the middle steak of the larger sized fish; one slice to weigh about 600 g (1¼ lb), this will make 4 good portions for grilling with butter. Being such a princely, pricey white fish, I think it is sacrilege to put halibut in a soup or stew, simple cooking is the answer. Bake in foil with a few fresh herbs or steam with herbs.

The largest halibut caught in British waters was 300 kg (660 lb) — I wonder who cooked that one for supper!

Halibut Steaks with Lemon Sauce

Serves 4

Ingredients

	Metric	Imperial	American
large steak of halibut cut through the middle	*600 g*	*1 ¼ lb*	*1 ¼ lb*
fresh dill			
leek, blanched part only, finely sliced	*1*	*1*	*1*
glass of dry white wine (Cinzano could be used)	*1*	*1*	*1*
seasoning to taste			
juice of lemon	*1*	*1*	*1*

Method

Place the fish in a shallow ovenproof dish so it sits on a bed of the dill and leek. Pour over the wine, add seasoning and lemon juice. Cover with a lid or foil. Bake in the oven at 180°C (350°F) Gas 4 for 10-15 minutes (this does depend on how thick the slice is). When testing, push the fork into the fish and gently pull to the side. The flesh should be almost firm, but not quite. If using a microwave, please double check the timing; it should be set at High and the fish cooked for no longer than 8 minutes. Serve with Lemon sauce (see page 17).

HERRING

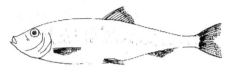

A pelagic — which means they like to swim in the upper levels of the sea, and they come in large shoals. Sad to think that 'once upon a time' they were so plentiful and cheap. However, they were overfished. Bans were imposed to allow the stocks to recover, and the herring fleets went out of business.

Now you know why we didn't see fresh herrings for so many years — in fact we forget all about them and certainly lost touch with what to do with them on the kitchen stove. In the olden days, especially just after World War II, salting, smoking, kippering, bloatering, buckling and sousing were all means of coping with the vast quantities. Although the herring is back in business and we have grown to appreciate those different methods of preservation, I can't ever see a time when we will be back to paying a couple of pence for 450 g (1 lb)! Yet today, herrings are still a fairly cheap food.

The humble herring is the most valuable fish of all our species. It certainly scores higher than any other fish in nutritional value. Herrings contain a good quantity of Vitamin D to help build bones in the young and old alike, Vitamin A for better eyesight and a healthy skin, packed with magic Eicosapentaenoic Acid (EPA) and Docosahexaenoic Acid (DHA) or OMEGA 3 —the wonder polyunsaturated oil that all dietitians and doctors are singing about today. A herring a day will surely keep the doctor away!

A herring can be recognized by its sparkling sea green back and streamlined shape, not usually longer the 30 cm (12 inches). Your fishmonger will always clean and trim for you but don't let him keep the roe, it is delicious on toast, especially the soft roe. You can roll fillets in oatmeal as everybody in Scotland will tell you. They can be grilled (no need for butter or oil) and are excellent cooked on the barbecue.

Welsh Herring Pie

Serves 3-4

Ingredients

	Metric	Imperial	American
herring fillets, thinly sliced	600 g	1¼ lb	1¼ lb
Dijon mustard	2 tbsp	2 tbsp	2 tbsp
seasoning to taste			
butter	50 g	2 oz	¼ cup
peeled potatoes	700 g	1½ lb	1½ lb
cooking apples, peeled and finely sliced	2	2	2
large onion, peeled and finely sliced	1	1	1
a little dried sage or finely chopped fresh sage			

Method

Flatten the herrings and spread with mustard. Season, then roll them up. Butter a pie dish, line with a layer of potato, apple, onion, finish off the butter and another layer of potato. Top with the herrings, sprinkle the sage over, then cover the dish. Bake in the oven 180°C (350°F) Gas 4 for 35 minutes. Cook for a further 15 minutes uncovered to crisp the potatoes, turning the herrings during this time. Serve with a green vegetable.

HERRING, MARINATED

A small Orkney cottage industry uses fresh-trawled herring and produces a tasty and delicious herring marinade base for smorgasboard or buffet menus — try herring marinade in fresh dill or sherry, with three other flavours to choose from. Loads of OMEGA 3.

HERRING ROE

The soft roe can be bought from a fishmonger separately, but it is usually frozen (all the leftovers from the kipper factory). If you buy 6 fresh herrings — watch what the fishmonger does with your roe. He won't know that you now know about dipping them in a little flour, frying in butter and serving on toast as a tasty supper dish!

HERRING, SMOKED   see Kippers, Bloaters, Buckling

HERRING, SOUSED

Sousing or spicing is vey suitable for oily fish. The acid in the marinade offsets the richness of the fish and softens those tiny bones — let children know that soused oily fish, including pilchards and mackerel, are very safe to eat without the use of a magnifying glass!

The marinade can be made up with cider, wine or vinegar, but don't use a coarse vinegar. A good red or white wine vinegar is worth the extra money.

Soused Herrings

Serves 4

Ingredients

	Metric	Imperial	American
herrings, filleted and beheaded	8	8	8
large Spanish onion, peeled and very thinly sliced	1	1	1
Marinade:			
3 parts vinegar to one part water/or mixture of wine and vinegar			
bay leaves	4	4	4
cloves	2	2	2
allspice	12	12	12
blades of mace	3	3	3
a pinch of salt			

Method

Roll up the fish, enclosing a little of the onion. Arrange in an ovenproof dish and cover with the marinade. Cover with foil and cook in the oven at 150°C (300°F) Gas 2 for 3-4 hours. When cooked, strain off the liquid and re-cover the herrings. Allow to go cold. Soused herrings will keep in the refrigerator for several days — they are delicious sliced into potato salad, topped with soured cream or fromage frais.

HUSS

Versatile in cooking; huss is also known as dogfish, flake and rigg. It is ideal for the short-sighted and children as it is cartilaginous,

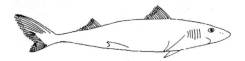

meaning non-bony. A meaty fish with a firm pinkish-white flesh, huss can be used for fish stew, soup, pie or fried in batter (Rock and Chips if you live in the South). Try sealing in a piece of foil with parsley, lemon and a bay leaf, cook in a moderate oven for 15-20 minutes (depending on the size). Serve with creamed potatoes amd mushy peas. If you find a huss on the end of your fishing line, don't attempt to skin it yourself — a machine is needed.

If you can't enjoy fish daily, feed the family with the capsules. For the record, 100,000 tons of cod liver oil were put into capsules last year!

JOHN DORY

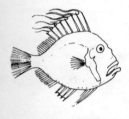

Such an ugly fish that when hauled from the Sea of Galilee, Saint Peter returned it to the water thinking it would frighten the children. The thumb prints of the Saint are to be seen to this day on each side of the fish. Despite its ugly, extremely large head, John Dory has a magnificent taste. Known as a 'Plymouth's proudest fish', large catches are landed at Newlyn in Cornwall. Choose a medium size fish, rub with butter and grill, then serve with lemon. Fillets can be taken from a large fish, your fishmonger will do this job for you, but ask for the head as well to make a good fish stock. If you fillet the fish yourself, you will find it easier to skin when cooked.

Poached John Dory

Serves 2

Ingredients

	Metric	Imperial	American
butter	*50 g*	*2 oz*	*¼ cup*
shallots, peeled and chopped	*2*	*2*	*2*
medium fillets John Dory, skinned	*4*	*4*	*4*
seasoned flour			
dry cider	*150 ml*	*¼ pint*	*⅔ cup*
fromage frais or natural yogurt mixed with a pinch of flour	*2 tbsp*	*2 tbsp*	*2 tbsp*
finely chopped fresh parsley to garnish			

Method

Melt the butter in a large frying pan and cook the shallots over a gentle heat for 3 minutes. Shake the fillets in flour, add to the pan with the cider and bring to the boil. Poach gently for 2 minutes. Lift out the fish on to warm plates. Quickly stir the fromage frais or yogurt into the pan — do not allow to boil. Serve immediately with the fish and a garnish of parsley.

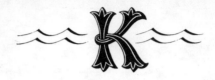

KING SCALLOPS
see Scallops and Queenies

General all year round availability from northern isles, subject to the weather. Available live in the shell or as shucked meat.

KIPPERS

A kipper is a fresh herring, cleaned, split down the back, given a brief soaking in brine and smoked for around 12 hours. If you happen to be in Fleetwood, you can send newly smoked Manx kippers to a friend in the South in a special box that will be delivered the following day — all things being equal. A good source of OMEGA 3 — a very tasty source as well. Try this idea if you don't want the smell of kippers at 7 in the morning:

Kippers in a Jug for Breakfast

Stand a pair of kippers in a heatproof jug, cover with boiling water and leave for 4 minutes. Perfect cooking — or you could stand it in an asparagus kettle if you have one!

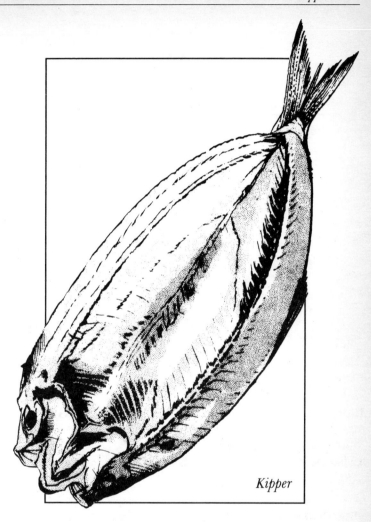

Kipper

Poor Man's Smoked Salmon

Allow boneless kippers to marinate in a vinaigrette made with wine vinegar, Dijon mustard, lemon juice and a little pepper. After a few hours, slice finely as for smoked salmon and enjoy with thin brown bread and butter.

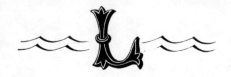

LEMON SOLE

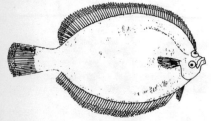

A member of the plaice family and should be cooked in the same way. Small ones can be grilled whole with a little butter as they are not one of the fatty fish. I was shown the finest of lemon soles by Ian Barlow when visiting the Brixham and Torbay Fish Company in Devon; and the locals confirmed what their choice was, compared to pricey Dover sole.

Devon Lemon Sole with Fresh Orange

Serves 2

Ingredients

	Metric	Imperial	American
large orange, plus a little extra orange juice	*1*	*1*	*1*

butter	50 g	2 oz	¼ cup
good size lemon sole, cut into fillets	1	1	1
flour	25 g	1 oz	¼ cup
seasoning to taste			
low fat or Gruyère cheese, grated	75 g	3 oz	¾ cup
finely chopped fresh parsley			

Method

Grate the rind from the orange reserving 2 slices for garnish. Squeeze out the juice and make up to 90 ml (3 fl oz/6 tbsp) with extra juice, then add sufficient water to make up to 200 ml (7 fl oz/⅞ cup).

Melt the butter in a frying pan with the orange rind and sauté for 2 minutes before adding the fish. Cook each side for 3 minutes, then lift into a gratin type dish to keep warm. To make the sauce, stir the flour into the pan and gradually add the orange juice. Season to taste, add the cheese to the smooth sauce, and stir continuously for 1 minute before pouring over the fish. Pop the dish under a hot grill for a few minutes to brown the top. Garnish with the parsley and slices of orange.

LING

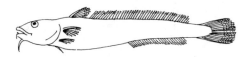

The largest member of the cod family, but not so good grilled or fried with chips. A true Yorkshire fish with ling pie being served from Filey to Saithes during Lent. A good fish for pie, soup, stew and the Chinese find ling very versatile for their methods of cooking.

Good Friday Pie with Mushy Peas

Serves 6

Ingredients

	Metric	Imperial	American
butter	25 g	1 oz	2 tbsp
flour	25 g	1 oz	¼ cup
milk, skimmed can be used	300 ml	½ pint	1¼ cups
chopped fresh parsley			
ling	700 g	1½ lb	1½ lb
large onion, peeled and chopped	1	1	1
hard-boiled eggs, roughly chopped	3	3	3
seasoning to taste			
ready made puff pastry	225 g	8 oz	½ lb

Method

Melt the butter in a pan and blend in the flour until smooth. Gradually add the milk, stirring continuously until smooth. Stir in the parsley. Place the fish in an ovenproof dish with the onion and egg. Top with sauce and seasoning.

Roll out the pastry to fit over the top of the dish, make two slits to allow air to escape. Pop in the oven at 220°C (425°F) Gas 7 and bake for 10 minutes and then reduce the heat to 180°C (350°F) Gas 4 and cook for a further 25 minutes until cooked through and the pastry is a nice golden brown. If you can be bothered it is worth brushing the pastry top with a little beaten egg and milk before cooking — depends who you are trying to impress! Serve with mushy peas.

LOBSTER

Still rather scarce in England unless you take your summer holidays in Cornwall and Devon — not to forget the Scottish Highlands and Islands.

As we all know, lobster has never been cheap, but then a fresh lobster caught around our British Isles has always been something special. However, the price will be coming down now that our shellfish boys are being inspired by the demand on the home front. Most of our fine catch ends up on gourmet tables in many countries — and they pay the price because they recognize 'quality'; the best Irish lobster I have only been able to enjoy at La Grappe D'Ore in Lausanne, Switzerland — cooked from live by Peter Baerman — lucky me!

But, if you ever find yourself 20 miles from Orford in Suffolk, time will not be wasted in a visit to The Oysterage. Bill Pinney not only farms his own Pacific (gigas) oysters for his restaurant all the year round, but between April and November he will present you with his own catch of fine lobster. Bill has certainly got the whole business of fish and shellfish together — and the tourists flock for miles. Julia Chapman from BBC Radio Suffolk and I encountered the most wonderful feasts of seafood when tripping around Suffolk seafood outlets with the UHA tape recorder — Bill's lobsters were exceptional.

And I still proclaim 'Hurray' for Maine and Canadian one and a half pounders, why not? I can enjoy lobster all the year round but please do the lobster a favour and keep away from anything frozen — a complete waste of time unless you have no appreciation for decent food.

And if you can't face cooking a live lobster, your friendly fishmonger will do this for you. Best to order a day in advance and arrange to collect when the fella is still warm (he will also cut it in two halves).

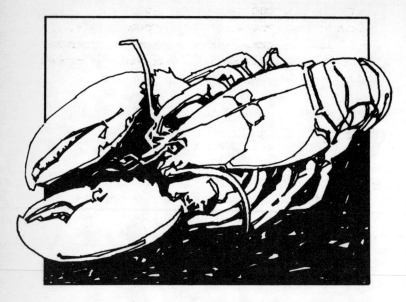

Get the nutcrackers ready to tackle the two front claws, half on each plate. Serve simply with a green salad, plenty of finely sliced cucumber and a little Wobbly mayonnaise (see page 16). If the lobster is for a special celebration enjoy the following dressing.

Brandy Dressing for Fresh Lobster

Mix the mayonnaise with a little fresh lemon juice and a good tot of brandy. Serve in a separate dish at the table.

or – the Shirly Fenugreek Special

Take 4 tablespoons real mayonnaise and mix with 4 tablespoons thick low-fat yoghurt. Mix in the juice of a lemon and a good measure of — wait for it — vodka! Combine well and then add finely powdered fenugreek — I add 1 teaspoon, but you can adjust according to your taste. Don't taste the lot and end up tipsy before you greet your guests!

Grilled Lobster

Serves 2

Ingredients

	Metric	Imperial	American
freshly cooked lobsters, about 500g(1lb 2oz) each, cut in halves	*2*	*2*	*2*
vegetable oil	*5 tbsp*	*5 tbsp*	*5 tbsp*
Worcestershire sauce	*3 tbsp*	*3 tbsp*	*3 tbsp*
clove of garlic, crushed	*1*	*1*	*1*
pinch of salt			
pinch of chopped fresh rosemary — or dried			
shake of pepper			

Method

Line the grill pan with foil and add the prepared lobster halves. Mix the remainder of the ingredients well and pour over the lobster. Cook under a fairly hot grill until lightly browned. Serve immediately with tiny new potatoes and a green salad.

Note: I sometimes sprinkle a little real freshly grated Parmesan cheese before grilling. However, I don't really advise to add anything that will deter from the distinctive and delicate flavour of a fresh lobster.

How to Prepare a Lobster

A Canadian or Maine lobster has a softer shell than a British or Irish lobster. It could be easier when preparing our own lobster catch to cut in half 'underside' because of the tougher shell — or involve your friendly fishmonger. A chef prefers to cut through as shown.

A sharp pointed knife will divide the lobster into two halves.

The two main claws contain superb white meat —have the nutcrackers at the ready to pass around to your guests.

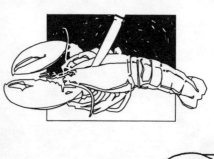

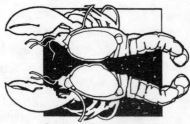

Drawings by Ray Liberty

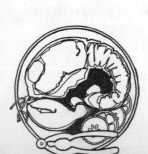

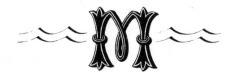

MACKEREL

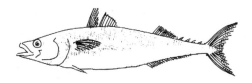

A pelagic fish which enjoys being one of a crowd, and there are plenty in the sea. You can stand on the sea shore in Cornwall and see shoals — all ready to jump on your plate for breakfast. A rich and oily fish with a firmer flesh than the herring, it must be eaten as fresh as possible. Don't buy if the eyes are suffering from a 'hangover', and the skin looks muggy and dull. Grill, fry, bake, marinade to souse. Can be potted, served hot or cold. A great source of OMEGA 3.

Grilled Very Fresh Mackerel

When dad comes home from his fishing trip with a basket of fresh mackerel — pick yourself a medium sized fish, chop off his head, slit along the belly to remove the innards and wash under the cold tap. Line the grill pan with foil, lay your fish on top and preheat the grill. Cook both sides for about 5-6 minutes, depending on size. Enjoy with a hunk of fresh brown bread and squeezes of fresh lemon.

MACKEREL, Smoked

The supermarkets are filled with smoked mackerel and they are quite delicious served cold with brown bread and butter. Try cutting into thin slices and serving with salad, or make a pâté to stuff into tiny vol-au-vent cases for a party.

Smoked Mackerel Pâté

Purée skinned smoked mackerel with equal amounts of cottage cheese or fromage frais, a little lemon juice and a few drops of Worcestershire sauce.

MEGRIM

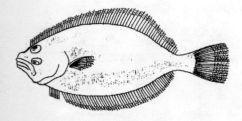

Megrim is one of the country cousins of the plaice family — a flat fish that can be grilled with a little butter. It is not too good poached or baked unless it has a good sauce to bring out a little more flavour. Ask your friendly fishmonger to fillet the fish for you; one fish will only be sufficient for one serving as fillets are not very plump.

MONKFISH Angler

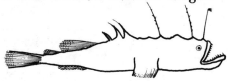

A deep water fish found off the coasts of Devon and Cornwall, although I have seen a few come up from Kent. Meaty when comparable to lobster and one of my favourites; it is a fish you can really get your teeth into. Watch out when trying 'scampi in the basket' on the South coast — it could be monkfish tails cut to the size of scampi and deep fried. Only the skinned tail is sold and there's very little wastage except for the huge ugly head. Poach with herbs and wine, or cook in foil with herbs and lemon. A great fish for kebabs cooked on the barbecue — just add chunks of pineapple, orange and mushrooms. Another useful fish for children as it has just one central bone.

Monkfish and Garlic

Serves 4

Ingredients

	Metric	Imperial	American
butter	*50 g*	*2 oz*	*¼ cup*
monkfish, filleted	*700 g*	*1½ lb*	*1½ lb*
chopped dill, tarragon and chives, mixed together			
ground black pepper			
cloves of garlic, crushed	*5*	*5*	*5*
button mushrooms, sliced	*100 g*	*4 oz*	*1 cup*
glass dry white wine	*1*	*1*	*1*
single cream or fromage frais	*4 tbsp*	*4 tbsp*	*4 tbsp*

Method

Butter a gratin dish well, lay the fillets of fish to fit across the base, then sprinkle over the herbs and pepper. Add the garlic and mushrooms, then pour over the wine. Cover and bake in the oven at 190°C (375°F) Gas 5 for 20 minutes. Lift the fish on to a serving dish. Fold the cream into the remaining liquid, pour over the fish and serve immediately.

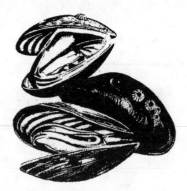

MUSSELS

Must be really fresh! You should have no problem if you have a reliable fishmonger. In bygone days when Molly Malone wheeled her wheelbarrow, there could have been a few doubtful molluscs in her basket! Purification treatment for farmed mussels is now obligatory. If you gather your own, only tread in clear waters — better to stick to your fishmonger who buys from a reliable source. When you get your fresh mussels home, toss into a bowl and store in the refrigerator (don't leave sealed in that plastic bag for days). They should be cooked within 24 hours. Scrub the mussels well, removing barnacles and beard, and discard any with cracked shells. Give a little tap to any that are open; if they don't close back immediately, they can also be discarded because they are dead. Always make sure that they are boiled for at least 2-3 minutes.

Cooked and shelled mussels are delicious with pasta and

Parmesan cheese, in a paella, a fish soup or stew, or cooked and cold with salt and vinegar. The easiest method, and favourite with everybody, must be the following:

Boiled Mussels with Garlic and Wine (Moules à la Marinière)

Serves 2

Ingredients

	Metric	Imperial	American
butter	*50 g*	*2 oz*	*¼ cup*
onion, peeled and finely chopped	*1*	*1*	*1*
cloves of garlic, chopped	*4*	*4*	*4*
dry white wine	*300 ml*	*½ pint*	*1¼ cups*
parsley, finely chopped (do not use dried)	*50 g*	*2 oz*	*2 oz*
black pepper			
fresh mussels, prepared	*1 kg*	*2 pints*	*5 cups*
grated Parmesan cheese (optional)	*50 g*	*2 oz*	*½ cup*

Method

In a large saucepan, melt the butter with the onion and garlic. Add the wine and half the parsley, plus a few turns of the black pepper mill. Cover the pan and simmer for 10 minutes. Add the prepared mussels to the pan. Cover, turn up the heat and cook for just 3 minutes — keep shaking the pan to distribute the mussels around. Turn into an ovenproof dish when all the mussels are open (discard any still tightly closed) with the stock. Sprinkle with the cheese, pop into a hot oven for 3 minutes. Garnish with parsley and enjoy with plenty of warm hunks of French bread. It is quite the

correct thing to dip your bread into the delicious juices
— and plenty of OMEGA 3.

However, if you visit Scotland, you will surely be
offered the wonderful 'Hanging Culture' farmed
mussel.

In the past people in Scotland thought of the wild
mussel as a natural and nutritious food and were
prepared to spend hours in a cold sea loch gathering
rough clumps for a 'rare feed' for the family. Today, that
flavour and value still remain, but it is no longer
necessary to scrape and clean the rough, barnacled
shells. The Scottish growers cultivate succulent shellfish
on ropes hanging freely in the unspoilt waters of the
Highlands and Islands. With a high meat content, the
farmed mussel is finding its rightful place in 'haute
cuisine'. The Belgo Restaurant, London NW1, is now
moving a ton of mussels a week — Molly Malone would
be green with envy.

Barbecued Farmed Mussels

With approximately 25 mussels to 1 kg (2 pints/5 cups)
— 'think' 12 mussels per person. Mix 2 crushed cloves
of garlic with plenty of fresh chopped parsley and a pot
of thick set natural yogurt or low-fat fromage frais.
Get the barbecue going until the charcoal glows.
Prepare the live mussels and place on the grid (a fish
slice could be useful for this job). I toss garlic onto the
charcoal — if nobody objects to garlic.
Lift the mussels as they open — this means they are
cooked — and divide around the guests who can help
themselves to cooked pasta and a helping of sauce.

And oysters cooked this way are magic!

Simple Mussel Salad
(With a few shrimps)

Serves 4-5

Ingredients

	Metric	Imperial	American
fresh mussels, prepared	2 kg	4-5 lb	4-5 lb
fish stock, can be made with stock cube	600 ml	1 pint	2½ cups
bunches watercress	4	4	4
virgin, cold pressed olive oil	120 ml	4 fl oz	½ cup
wine vinegar	2 tbsp	2 tbsp	2 tbsp
seasoning to taste			
fresh cooked pink or brown shrimps, without heads	225 g	8 oz	1⅓ cups
large red pepper, deseeded and chopped	1	1	1
spring onions, chopped (chives could be used)	4	4	4

Method

Cook the mussels in the stock until all the shells have opened, about 4 minutes. Remove the meat from the shells.

Remove the thick stalks from the watercress (save these for a watercress soup). Mix the oil and vinegar with seasoning. Mix all the ingredients together and chill for 30 minutes before serving.

OYSTERS

I don't care what noise annoys an oyster most — my favourite sound is that knife scraping apart the shell and opening up a delicious prospect.

Ned Sherrin

Still very much recognised as a sound love potion or 'aphrodisiac'. Buy six for a starter and see!

Now I have encouraged everybody back into the oyster habit, be assured that they are now safe to enjoy all the year round — so there's no need to resist temptation 'til there's an 'R' in the month. This belief was based on laws governing the harvest of the native (edulis) oyster — these now command a high price as demand exceeds supply. The salvation for all oyster addicts must be the farmed Pacific (gigas) oyster, which is now grown in some of the most beautifully remote regions around the British Isles, available all year round at an affordable price.

An oyster knife is undoubtably a good investment; and the Rossmore oyster cracker is magic. Although your fishmonger will always do the opening for you. Once you get the knack, the job is easy and don't waste a drop of that precious juice.

Ask your friendly fishmonger to order your oysters if he doesn't already carry a continuous supply. Watch out for oysters at larger supermarkets with a wet fish counter.

Freezing oysters could not be easier and so there's no reason now why anybody couldn't keep a supply in their own home. The shell gapes slightly when they are thawed making them easier to open for the less experienced oyster addict. (Allow 1 hour at least to thaw and consume swiftly.)

Many 'oysteries' throughout the UK are sending fresh oysters daily by overnight courier service to anywhere in the UK mainland. Bountiful supplies are to be had from the shores of Seasalter (Whitstable) to the Lochs of Scotland drifting to Wales and Northern Ireland — British oysters delivered to your door. Now the famous Dorset native (edulis) not only sweeping through oyster bars in the UK, but also sweeping through top restaurants in Switzerland and Germany, not to forget Monte Carlo. And thinking oyster bars, I wonder how many people in the business know the original Wheelers still survives in Whitstable. I remember Ned Sherrin, (who is certainly a great 'oyster aficianado') quoting that the finest oysters he had ever tasted came from under Delia's counter in Whitstable. Delia can produce both Native and Pacific oysters directly from her very own purification tank at Seasalter Shellfish (Whitstable) Ltd.

1. Hold the oyster in a cloth, placing cup side in palm of hand firmly.

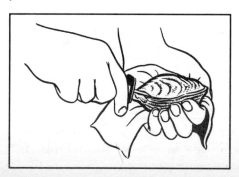

2. The experts in London prefer to insert the knife at the hinge — I was taught by a French doctor to go into the oyster at the side (the side where you find the muscle). See the drawing and take your pick.

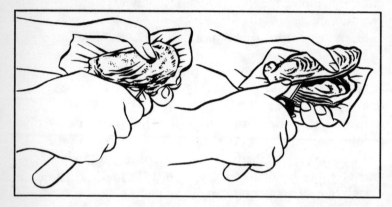

3. Take seconds and care to see the dividing line for the two halves of shell, pierce through, gently severing top muscle from the oyster — keep the oyster level not to lose the precious juice — once pierced through, the top shell will come away with ease.

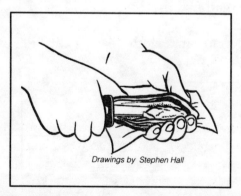

Drawings by Stephen Hall

4. Slide the knife to gently sever bottom muscle. The oyster meat will now flow from the shell.

OYSTER KNIFE Do invest in a decent knife, a cheapie one will bend and rust. Not too wide a blade as some Swiss chefs prefer; not too pointed a tip to mutilate the oyster flesh. Ladies, watch for the new 'oyster cracker'. This wonderful new invention does work well, and if the wrist feels a little under par, it certainly takes away any strain — and it is very safe.

Frozen Oysters on Beds of Spinach

Serves 2

Every time you indulge in fresh oysters at home, save a few until you have a dozen in the freezer — they do freeze quite well. For a very easy supper dish to make for a romantic evening, try the following.

Ingredients

	Metric	Imperial	American
Packet of frozen spinach or 450g (1 lb) fresh, cooked	1	1	1
Pacific oysters from the freezer	12	12	12
butter	50 g	2 oz	¼ cup
grated nutmeg			

Method

Thaw the spinach. Pass the spinach through a food processor to purée. The oysters will take about 1 hour to thaw at cool room temperature and they will also open themselves.

Remove the oysters from the shells and toss in a little butter gently over medium heat for 2 minutes. Arrange the spinach on 2 serving plates, then add the oysters. Garnish with a little grated nutmeg.

Things Ain't What They Used To Be!

Oysters for Xmas Gifts

The kits are beautifully made of thick, solid oak, elegantly finished off with two broad gilded hoops. They measure 12 inches in diameter, and 6 inches deep, and after use can be turned into decorative garden ornaments.

CONTENTS OF KIT

1. Four Dozen **Selected Whitstable Oysters.**
2. An Oyster Opener.
3. Instructions how to open, and how to keep Oysters; and particulars of the wonderful properties of Oysters.

Each kit is despatched wrapped in cellophane (to keep it clean) and packed in wooden case to ensure safe transit.

Carriage Paid Price 23/6 each.

A similar KIT with Four Dozen Extra Selected

BLUEPOINTS - 17/6

All you need do is . . . .
1. Send us your own addressed labels, with any Greeting Cards to be enclosed.
2. Mention date you wish them delivered. The Kits will be delivered to any address **CARRIAGE PAID.**

Orders should be given as early as possible. If orders are delayed we cannot guarantee dispatch as it is impossible to have additional kits Coopered at short notice.

- -

HAROLD CAYLESS

Fish & Poultry Specialist,

2 & 63 Goodmayes Road, GOODMAYES, Essex.

Telephone: Seven Kings 1800 & 3100.

ORDER FORM

Please Supply:-

.... *Kit(s) of Whitstable Oysters.*

.... *Kit(s) of Bluepoint Oysters.*

and forward to the following address:— (in Block letters)

....

....

to arrive on December ...., 1937.

Yours faithfully,

An order form for oysters dating back to 1937.

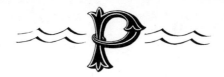

PIKE

A freshwater fish often caught by fishermen in rivers and ponds. Best to use in a pie, soup or a stew, and the liver is considered a delicacy. Its claim to fame must be as Quenelles (very fattening fish dumplings that the French adore). My advice is to throw the fella straight back from whence he came!

PILCHARDS (Adult Sardines)

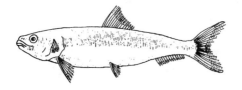

If you go anywhere near Cornwall you will learn that pilchards don't all get fished out of the sea in a tin. One of the most famous oily fish that are laced with OMEGA 3. Similar to the herring and mackerel, pilchards can therefore be cooked in the same way. The following pie is traditional in Cornwall and it looks so pretty when served — it can also be made with large sardines and herrings.

Stargazy Pie

Serves 4-5

Arrange cleaned fresh pilchards in an ovenproof dish, the heads should be over the side of the dish. Add chopped onion, hard-boiled eggs and plenty of chopped parsley and seasoning to taste. Add a few sea vegetables, about 25 g(1 oz) to make a feast. Top with a pastry crust. Bake in the oven at 180°C (350°F) Gas 4 for about 35-40 minutes.

PLAICE

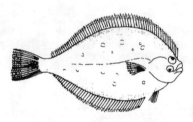

In Herne Bay, Kent, I bought 1.5 kg (3 lb) for 80p — who said that fish was expensive? Don't be put off by small plaice, they are simply delicious popped under a grill with a painting of butter and served with a squeeze of lemon — no need to go into the performance with batter. If, by chance, you do get a real whopper, then you can fillet, roll in egg and breadcrumbs, deep fry and serve with chips — oven cooked for better health of course! Whatever way you decide to cook, you can't go wrong when the plaice is so cheap.

POLLACK

A relative of the cod family recognized by its slightly yellowish sides. Use in the same way as any of the solid white fish in casseroles, soups or pies; a fish with very little fat, it therefore needs a little juice or sauce.

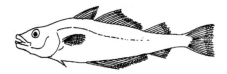

Pollack with Mustard Sauce

Spread steaks of pollack with mild Dijon mustard. Shallow fry both sides in butter or groundnut oil. When cooked, lift on to a serving plate and keep warm. Shake a little flour into the frying pan, stir in a glass of dry white wine and a little chopped parsley or fresh thyme. Keep stirring and add some cream, season to taste. To serve, pour the sauce over the fish and have a few new potatoes and peas at the ready.

PRAWNS

Prawns, prawns, what is a prawn? Or is it a shrimp? We don't find too many of the obvious prawns in our waters. I mean the big ones that are red when they are caught and stay red when they are boiled — they usually arrive in our kitchen frozen from Greenland or Norway.

These cold water prawns benefit from growing more slowly than the 'warm water' variety that come from India and the Far East which have a decidedly 'woolly' texture. The Greenland prawn, in particular, takes years to grow in temperatures that are just above freezing. The resulting flavour of these prawns is thought by many to be the best in the world. So, a plea, *don't* use cold water prawns for cooking — leave that for the warm water prawns.

We do have a few of the smaller variety which are colourless and turn pink on boiling — and these have the better flavour. If you can buy the fresh, they are delicious grilled with a little chopped garlic in butter. Serve as a starter with a little Lemon mayonnaise (see page 17). It is correct to eat with the fingers, simply pick off the heads, open the shells from underneath and pull away. Don't forget brown bread and butter and the finger bowls.

Prawn Cocktail

Here is a new look for a traditional favourite — and much healthier too!

Serves 4

Ingredients

	Metric	Imperial	American
iceberg lettuce and raddiccio, finely shredded			
cooked and peeled prawns, thawed	225 g	8 oz	1⅓ cups
lemon juice			
mint sprigs to garnish	4	4	4
Sauce:			
plain thick Greek yogurt	100 g	4 oz	½ cup
juice of lemon	½	½	½
clove of garlic, crushed	½	½	½
handful of mint leaves, roughly chopped, or diced cucumber			
seasoning to taste			

Method

Layer the lettuce in the bases of 4 wine or Champagne glasses. Pile 50 g (2 oz/⅓ cup) prawns on each, moisten with a little lemon juice.

Mix together the yogurt, lemon juice and garlic and mint or cucumber, then season well. Mask the top prawns generously with the sauce and garnish with a sprig of mint on each cocktail.

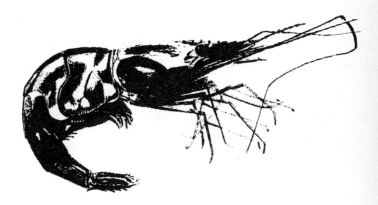

Prawn

PRINCESS SCALLOPS   see Scallops and Queenies

Delicious smoked from Benesther Shellfish, Orkney (winner of 1989 'Food From Britain' best smoked seafood competition).

QUEENIES

These are much smaller than a scallop but all from the same family. They are best between November and March.

Queenies in Fromage Frais Sauce

Serves 2

Ingredients

	Metric	Imperial	American
noodles	225 g	8 oz	½ lb
fromage frais	2 tbsp	2 tbsp	2 tbsp
soured cream	2 tbsp	2 tbsp	2 tbsp
juice of lemon	1	1	1
finely chopped chives	2 tbsp	2 tbsp	2 tbsp
seasoning to taste			
queenies	10	10	10

Method

Cook the noodles and keep warm. Mix the fromage frais with the soured cream, lemon juice, chives and seasoning to taste. To cook the queenies, cover in boiling water and allow to stand for 1 minute only. (NO, you can't use your microwave because it is too quick and will overcook all scallops.) Drain the queenies, mix into the sauce and spoon over the noodles.

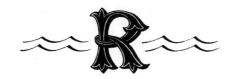

RAY

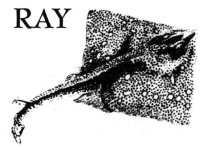

A skate, thornbac, torpedo or kindred flat-bodied elasmobranch fish (to quote the English dictionary). You will usually find the fish has been prepared and just the large wings are available. If you catch a ray fish, don't eat it for at least 2 days after catching when the flavour will be better. Cook as for Skate.

RED MULLET

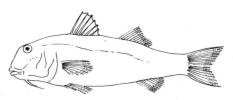

Can be treated as grey mullet, although it is a superior fish. Plenty to be found around the South Coast. Like grey mullet, this is a very bony fish — not advisable to feed it to very young children.

With older children, looking for bones in fish can be fun. Encourage them to have a go at setting every bone they find around the plate — then you can all sing 'Tinker, Tailor, Soldier, Sailor' — well it does encourage children to eat more fish. Plenty of OMEGA 3 for everybody.

Red Mullet in a Parcel

Serves 1

Ingredients

	Metric	Imperial	American
medium red mullet	1	1	1
lemon slices	5	5	5
chopped parsley			
knob of butter			
a little white pepper and pinch of salt			

Method

Wash the fish, removing the scales. Clean the mullet, see Note. Seal the fish in foil with the ingredients. Cook in the oven at 180°C (350°F) Gas 4 for 15-20 minutes. Enjoy with creamed or new potatoes and a side salad.

Note: To clean a round fish, slit along the belly using a knife. Using the fingers or a knife remove the innards; reserve the roe of red mullet, it is a great delicacy. Rinse the fish under cold water.

RIGG   see Huss

ROE   see Cod's Roe and Herring Roe.
Laced with OMEGA 3, especially the cod roe.

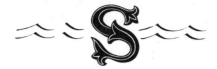

SAITHE   see Coley

SALMON

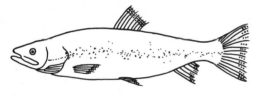

Wild salmon can still be caught in our British
rivers and estuaries in season. The introduction
of salmon farming, however, has meant that this glorious
product is now available fresh all year round.

So popular is salmon these days that salmon farming
production now exceeds the total output of beef in the
Highlands of Scotland; indeed, over 36000 tonnes of
farmed Scottish salmon was produced in 1991 of which at
least 30000 tonnes ended up on the fishmongers' slab or in
the supermarket in the UK — and it has plenty of
OMEGA 3.

'Be not afraid; be prepared!'

Raw salmon smoked is a great delicacy throughout the
world but for real connoisseurs there's nothing quite like
the true flavour of fresh salmon. To appreciate the delicate
flavour of fresh salmon be sure you do not overcook. Look

for Scottish salmon symbol when buying your fresh salmon — the market will soon be flooded with salmon from as far afield as Canada, Norway and Greenland; and all good stuff. But there is nothing to compare with the quality and flavour of our own Highland and Island salmon — and always take my first choice from the Shetland Isles (marked Atlantic) if you have a choice; a little extra boost added to the feed, but guaranteed purity to the last slice.

Cooking for one or twenty, fresh salmon is so easy to prepare and adaptable — grilled, boiled or baked or poached whole fish. A 150g (5 oz) serving makes a substantial meal for one, and think how many 150 g (5 oz) servings you will get from a whole salmon. It can't be called expensive food when you consider the low price of a whole farmed salmon today.

Baked Salmon

Dill is my favourite herb for this recipe. Don't use the dried variety; if no fresh herbs are available, just use a little seasoning and a few slices of lemon. A dried bay leaf could also be used.

Serves 8 with a little to spare

Ingredients

	Metric	Imperial	American
fresh salmon, cleaned	*2.5 kg*	*5-6 lb*	*5-6 lb*
lemon, cut into slices	*1*	*1*	*1*
fresh dill, tarragon, parsley			
* or mint*			

Method

Don't bother to remove the scales, together with the skin they help to keep a whole fish in good shape during cooking. Seal the fish with a few slices of lemon and fresh herbs (you can mix the lot together) in foil. Stand on a tray or roasting dish and cook on the middle shelf of the oven at 180°C (350°F) Gas 4, allowing 6-7 minutes for each 450 g (1 lb), plus 15 minutes. Cooking time is really a matter of personal taste. Some people prefer the fish to be slightly undercooked while others like everything 'well done'. Just don't go away and leave the salmon in the oven for hours — it will be like rubber when you get back!

Remove from the oven then allow to stand for 10 minutes before peeling off the skin (start from the head end using the blunt side of a knife) from the top side and fins. Lift on to a serving plate using the foil as a hoist, split the foil at both ends and lift to ease from under the fish. Serve warm with new potatoes and peas, plus Wobbly mayonnaise (see page 16) and a hint of lemon.

If you really want to impress and display the whole fish at the table, arrange thinly sliced cucumber (don't peel) down the middle of the skinned fish.

SALMON, SMOKED

Exactly what it states, raw smoked salmon, cut in wafer thin slices. Serve with fresh lemon juice, black pepper and brown bread and butter for a special occasion. It is almost traditional to have smoked salmon and scrambled eggs for Christmas Day breakfast — for extra treats.

SALMON TROUT

There is no such fish. You will frequently see a sea trout (even a large brown trout) labelled 'salmon trout' — it's a bit unfair of a fishmonger or restaurateur to try and pull a fast one to obtain a higher price. A sea trout is a very fine fish in its own right, with a fine delicate flavour. Cook as for salmon. Plenty of OMEGA 3.

SARDINES

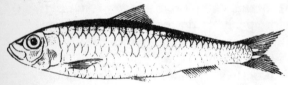

An oily fish that is a pelagic (see page 67). Grilled all over the world and cheap. I just wish that we could find a few more of the fresh variety on our fishmonger's slab. Sardines do enjoy some of our British waters, although the mass come from Portugal and Spain in a tin. The South coast of Ireland is another catching ground and, if we have a heatwave, shoals can be found in the North Sea. The moral must be; if you see fresh sardines — buy them and give the family a treat.

Cook them on the barbecue straight out of the sea, or toss in seasoned flour and fry in a little groundnut oil. Serve with fresh lemon.

Sardines are never too expensive and yet they are packed with such great nutritional value — OMEGA 3, plenty of iron and calcium. And don't under estimate those little tins of sardines! Premenopausal, the menopause and OSTEO-

POROSIS are now familiar names to women reaching that exciting age. Calcium for bone loss! One tin of sardines (with the bones) is a better source of calcium than all your pills in a jar — and tastier. Mash a whole tin of sardines with the bones, plus a dash of cider vinegar, to top hot toast for a solo supper.

SCALLOPS (King, Princess)

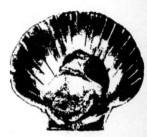

Like queenies but larger in size. Molluscs with such a delicate flavour — but they are not cheap. I have enjoyed fresh scallops when on holiday in Devon and Cornwall. (I don't consider the frozen version to be in the same class.) The price is high because they don't like travelling — unlike an oyster. Where the oyster will keep himself fairly insular for many days, once out of the purification tanks the scallop gives in and opens his shell after about 12 hours. One consolation is that a little goes a long way. Four fresh scallops will give sufficient flavour to a mousse for four portions; one poached in the shell with a rich cheese topping makes an excellent starter.

Scallops

Allow 2 scallops per person. To prepare, first remove the red coral and set aside. Discard the black vein and muscle from the side of the body. Slice the remaining parts and fry over a gentle heat in butter for 2 minutes.

Add the coral and cook for a further minute. Serve with warm wholemeal toast. There is plenty of OMEGA 3 in the coral.

SEA BASS

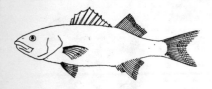

This very fine fish is the very special prize for the West Country angler — can be found occasionally in fresh water from spring to autumn. Not a cheap fish, but worth every penny if you are lucky enough to find one on the fishmonger's slab. A round fish that can weigh from 2.5-7 kg (5-16 lb). There are only two respectful ways to cook this beautiful fish — on a barbecue on the beach or bake for a party if your Premium Bonds come up!

Baked Sea Bass for a Party

Serves 8

Ingredients

	Metric	Imperial	American
sea bass, descaled and cleaned	3 kg	6½ lb	6½ lb
softened butter	75 g	3 oz	6 tbsp
cloves of garlic, crushed	5	5	5
plenty of fresh rosemary			
seasoning to taste			

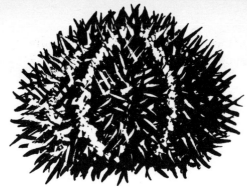

Sea Urchin

Method

Stuff the fish with half the butter, the garlic and rosemary. Season. Brush the skin with the remaining butter and seal the whole fish in foil. Bake in the oven at 190°C (375°F) Gas 5 for 25-35 minutes depending how well you like it cooked. Serve with new potatoes, and wedges of lemon.

SEA BREAM   see Bream

SEA URCHINS

Found on the Irish and South West English coastlines and a few parts of Scotland; with masses ready to invade our markets from Norway. Many that are caught in British waters are packed off immediately to France where they are very much appreciated for their delicate orange coloured ovaries that are eaten raw with lemon juice and black pepper. I think I prefer my sea urchins cooked, like egg, with plenty of real mayonnaise and fresh lemon juice. Please note well; no doubt because they have a high zinc and iron content they are excellent as a hang-over cure: plenty of OMEGA 3 too.

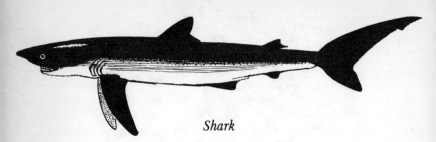

Shark

SHARK

The most popular found in British waters is the tope or
porbeagle with its pinkish firm flesh and excellent flavour.
(Other species have white meat.) If you do buy a steak of
shark, just grill with a little knob of butter and shake of
pepper and salt. Serve with a squeeze of lemon juice — all
quite delicious and exciting. See also Tope.

SHRIMPS

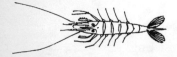

Brown potted shrimps and Morecombe Bay go together
like mustard and cress. Having been born on the sands of
Blackpool myself, I am bound to state that the finest little
crustaceans are to be purchased anywhere on the Fylde
coastline. Potted in butter or eaten straight from the paper
carton with plenty of buttered Hovis with a dash of vinegar
and a shake of the pepper pot — they are superb. Shrimps
are boiled immediately on the boat when caught because
they don't keep well. Although it does not happen in the
UK, many countries have huge factories where the shrimps

are actually peeled immediately they come off the boats. What bliss. Have you ever tried peeling a pound of shrimps in a hurry for tea?

SHRIMPS, PINK

These are transparent pink when raw and can be eaten whole when cooked. Tropical shrimps (thanks to farming) are now becoming big business in our import market.

It is better for the waistline and far more interesting to sit and watch telly eating fresh shrimps, be they brown or pink, rather than a bag of boiled sweets. Just keep a separate little pot to hold the heads and tails as you pick them off so quickly. The children will love them too.

SKATE

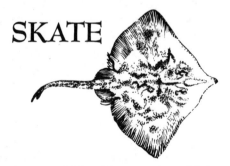

A very odd looking species of fish — it looks as though it has just arrived from outer space. You may see a whole fish on a special display, but on the fishmonger's slab you will only see the pinky coloured, ready skinned, wings. It's all quite delicious, especially if you find the knob — you know that tasty little bit on a chicken (that nestles between the leg and the backbone on each side) — skate knobs are the jaw muscle of the fish and remind me of the same part. Skate can be poached with a few fresh herbs and butter, grilled, or deep fried with a coating of batter. The bones are more like gristle and won't frighten the children.

Fried Skate Wings with Fresh Lemon

Cut the wings into manageable pieces. Dip in seasoned flour and fry lightly in butter and oil. Serve with wedges of lemon.

Skate Knob Kebabs

Although popular, scallops can be scarce and expensive. Skate knobs, on the other hand, are delicious, cheap and not thought about very often. You have to fiddle a bit to remove any gristly bone and sort out a thick kebab to stick on a skewer, bedded in a small piece of cheese. A little seasoning is all that is needed before grilling on the barbecue, popping under the grill, or frying in a pan coated with a little rape seed oil (turn during cooking time). If you feel like being a little 'exotic' — roll in Pesto sauce before cooking. Cooking time would be around 4 minutes — all depends on the size of the skate knobs. Delicious and interesting.

Note: If you are searching for your skate knobs in the East End of London you should ask for 'Eye Balls'. Yes, correct name for delicious skate knobs. I have it on good authority that they are delicious boiled and served with parsley sauce.

SMELTS

A little fish (for some strange reason smelling of cucumber) that is cooked whole under the grill and is excellent strung on to skewers with mushrooms and fruit (pineapple, peaches, plums or apple) — making great kebabs!

SOLE   see Dover Sole and Lemon Sole

SPRATS

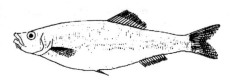

Another tiny fish, sometimes mistaken for a baby herring — well it is a member of the same family. Southwold and Aldeburgh take claim as having the finest catch through the winter months. They are very nutritious and contain plenty of OMEGA 3.

Vera's Fried Sprats

Wash fish well and sprinkle with a little sea salt. Get a frying pan nice and hot — no fat needed — and fry the fish quickly, turning during the cooking time. The salt will bring out all the fat needed to keep the fish moist and tasty. Serve with fresh lemon juice.

SQUID

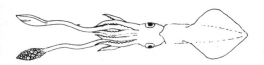

Well we certainly eat plenty of squid when on holiday abroad — Tapas in Spain, with pasta in Italy, the Greeks deep fry and the French add squid to anything 'Fritto

Misto'. Cuttlefish can be cooked the same way. Your fishmonger will always do the basic preparation of removing eye section and intestine, but it is easy to remove any tough cartilage type membrane from the neck that might be left. A thin bone runs the length of the fish, loosen slightly at the top, then ease out holding body. Rub the red and black spotted layer from the body under running cold water, and do the same with the tentacles. Alternatively, it's easy to find prepacked and frozen in the supermarket. Cooking time must either be short or long; anything in between will make the texture like rubber.

Fritto Misto to Cook at Home

Serves 4

Ingredients

	Metric	Imperial	American
mixed squid or cuttlefish and any other solid white fish	700 g	1½ lb	1½ lb
Batter:			
plain flour	2 tbsp	2 tbsp	2 tbsp
half milk and half water	150 ml	¼ pint	⅔ cup
egg white	1	1	1

Method

For the batter, blend the flour into the milk and water. Allow to stand for 1 hour before using, then beat in the egg white.

Cut the prepared fish into small pieces and cut the squid in thin rings. Toss the fish in flour, dip in the batter and deep fry for about 3-4 minutes.

Saffron Squid

This recipe uses the body and tentacles together.

Serves 3-4

Ingredients

	Metric	Imperial	American
large onion, peeled and finely sliced	1	1	1
cloves garlic, chopped	2	2	2
virgin cold pressed olive oil	1 tbsp	1 tbsp	1 tbsp
large red pepper, deseeded and sliced	1	1	1
strands of saffron soaked in 1 cup of boiling water	5	5	5
squid, cleaned and cut in bite size pieces	1	1	1
white wine	1 cup	1 cup	1 cup
seasoning to taste			

Method

Sauté the onion and garlic in the oil for 4 minutes over gentle heat. Add the red pepper and saffron with water, then simmer with the pan covered for 4 minutes. Add squid and wine to the pan with seasoning to taste, cover and simmer for 7-8 minutes having given the ingredients a good stir. When cooked, serve on a bed of long grain rice.

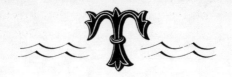

TOPE *see also Shark*

Can be used as Cod. A good firm flesh that can be cubed and grilled for kebabs. It's cheaper than cod, better than rock eel and has no bones, only cartilage like gristle so it is easy for children to eat.

TROUT

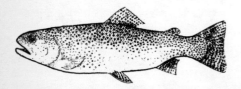

Almost all trout eaten in the British Isles today is farmed. This is all great news because we can now indulge in this vey fine fish all the year round. With trout, you can bake, fry, grill, microwave, devil, make fishcakes, omelettes, even a risotto. What's more, trout is really laced with nutritional value — plenty of OMEGA 3 and the price is right.

You won't find too many brown trout on the table, today they are farmed for restocking angling rivers, lakes and ponds. The rainbow trout is ideal for farming because it grows so quickly wherever there is an abundant supply of cool, clear and pure water. As for salmon trout, there is no such species: the terminology has been invented by the catering trade to command a better price on a large trout.

Poached Trout with Tangy Mayonnaise

Serves 2

Ingredients

	Metric	Imperial	American
fresh trout, cleaned with heads and tails left on	2	2	2
Wobbly mayonnaise (see page 16)	4 tbsp	4 tbsp	4 tbsp
natural low-fat yogurt	6 tbsp	6 tbsp	6 tbsp
juice of lime or lemon	1	1	1
watercress to garnish			

Method

Clean the fish under the cold running tap, trim the tail to a nice 'V' shape. Place in an ovenproof dish, cover with cold water, then foil. Cook in the oven at 180°C (350°F) Gas 4 for 20 minutes — the trout will be cooked when the eyes become white and opaque. If you are cooking a large fish, skin the cooked fish, (still with head and tail intact), which is easy while the fish is still warm. Remove the eyes and leave until cold.

Mix the mayonnaise with the yogurt and lime juice and serve in a separate dish. Garnish the whole fish with watercress.

To serve the trout hot: cook and prepare as before, pop on to warm plates and serve with garlic butter — you can now find it ready prepared in the supermarket.

Note: If you really can't stand the sight of a fish head on your plate — perhaps the children are not too keen — trout fillets are now readily available. Trout fillets have a few pin-bones only, which can't do great harm.

Fisherman's Trout — Cooked the Poacher's Way

Tickle your trout on to the river bank, wrap tightly in a soaking wet tabloid newspaper (only tabloid less than a day old will do). Cook in a Dutch oven made of bricks, on the river bank, until the paper is dry. No need for plates, fingers were invented before knives and forks. No fishy cooking smells in the open air.

TROUT, SEA

Spring is the best season for a sea trout, known as Sewin in West Wales. Treat yourself to a three pounder and cook as salmon.

A sea trout is a relative of the salmon that migrates to estuaries and other inshore waters to search for food. The richer diet and warm waters cause rapid growth and the fish matures into a pink fleshed fish with a wonderful flavour.

Please don't curry, stew, soup or fry — just cook with 'loving care' like a poached or baked salmon.

TROUT, SMOKED

Plain or peppered, both can be found in the supermarket and every delicatessen counter. Serve with soured cream and wedges of lemon. Cut into 2.5 cm (1 inch) strips and toss into a mixed salad. Alternatively, pop in the food processor with cream, yogurt, nutmeg and black pepper — wonderful dip or filling for vol-au-vents.

TUNA

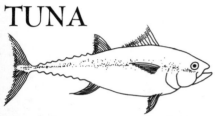

The only way to use fresh tuna is to grill it —delicious. Never buy the frozen because it is horrid! —tinned is better.

Tuna Mousse

Serves 4

Ingredients

	Metric	Imperial	American
gelatine	*15 g*	*½ oz*	*½ oz*
tomato juice	*300 ml*	*½ pint*	*1¼ cups*
tins of tuna in brine	*1-2*	*1-2*	*1-2*
(different brands vary in weight) about 295g(10oz/10oz)			
finely chopped fresh parsley	*1 tbsp*	*1 tbsp*	*1 tbsp*
black pepper to taste			

Method

Make up the gelatine with a little water as instructed on the packet to set the tomato juice. Purée all the ingredients in a blender or food processor. Alternatively, chop the fish very well and fold into the tomato juice with the remaining ingredients. Whatever method you use, turn the tuna and tomato mixture into a mould and allow to set. Serve in slices with cucumber and radishes.

Tuna Salad for One

Serves 1

Ingredients

	Metric	Imperial	American
tin of tuna in natural juice, about 185g(6oz/6oz)	1	1	1
shallot or spring onion, finely chopped	50 g	2 oz	½ cup
small red pepper, finely chopped	1	1	1
clove of garlic, crushed	1	1	1
hard-boiled egg, chopped	1	1	1
Wobbly mayonnaise (see page 16)	1 tbsp	1 tbsp	1 tbsp
shredded salad to serve			

Method

Drain the fish well and flake. Mix with the remainder of the ingredients and serve piled high on a bed of shredded salad. Black olives look so pretty for a garnish.

Tuna with Brown Rice

Serves 4

Ingredients

	Metric	Imperial	American
small onions or shallots, peeled and finely chopped	2	2	2
cloves of garlic, finely chopped	2	2	2
olive oil	1 tbsp	1 tbsp	1 tbsp
brown rice	150 g	5 oz	⅔ cup
stock made with Vecon or vegetable cube	300 ml	½ pint	1¼ cups
tomatoes, peeled and chopped	3	3	3
a little black pepper			
a few strands of saffron			
tins of tuna in natural juice, about 295g (10oz/10oz), drained	1-2	1-2	1-2
tin sweetcorn, drained well	220 g	8 oz	8 oz
chives to garnish			

Method

Sauté the onions and garlic in the oil for 4 minutes. Add the rice and allow to cook with the onion for 3 minutes, stirring continuously. Pour in the stock, tomatoes, pepper and saffron. Cover and simmer for at least 35 minutes or until the rice is tender. Add the tuna and sweetcorn, then heat gently for a further 10 minutes. Garnish with a few chopped chives.

TURBOT

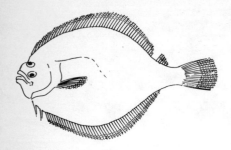

Found in the North Sea, a big fish from the flat fish family. Sold in steaks or fillets, it is an expensive fish with an exquisite flavour not to be spoilt with exotic sauces and too many trimmings — just simplicity. Popular on the Christmas menu or for a special occasion, a large turbot can weigh anything up to 20 kg (45 lb) but you can find one or two chicken turbots at around 1 kg (2½ lb) to cook whole. It can be cooked in foil with a bay leaf and slices of lemon. Alternatively, in milk, a 250 g (9 oz) steak will take about 8 minutes to poach. Remove the skin when cooked.

Poached turbot, left to cool a little to be decorated for a fish buffet, will show what a very gelatinous fish it is. Not only an oily fish but still packed with plenty of goodness and protein.

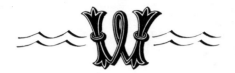

WHELKS

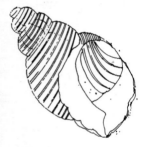

Off the Kent coast at Whitstable, the whelk boats bring their catch in baskets to the harbour sheds, and the ladies still sit in a circle and shell the cooked molluscs by hand.

The older generation still love to chew through their tough old whelks with their false teeth — I like to chop them up in a food processor, mix with mayonnaise and spread on toast.

I have it on very good authority that Wells-Next-the-Sea in Norfolk, supplies 80% of all whelks sold today.

WHITEBAIT

The tiny silver fry (young) of the herring. Shoals are caught in large nets around the Wash between June and October, where you

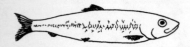

will find plenty in the local cafes and restaurants. Come September and October, you will have to go fishing further down south to Southend and catch the Whitebait Festival — although daft as it may seem, all the whitebait at this time are frozen. For a little bit of fishy history, whitebait parties were held to celebrate the end of Parliament in the 19th century.

Oven Cooked Whitebait

Loads of OMEGA 3.

Serves 2

Ingredients

	Metric	Imperial	American
butter or oil for greasing			
fresh or frozen whitebait, dredged in seasoned flour	450 g	1 lb	1 lb

Method

Cover a baking tray with foil and grease well with butter or oil. Sprinkle out the whitebait on the tray. Bake in the oven at 200°C (400°F) Gas 6 for about 15 minutes. Serve immediately with wedges of lemon and newly baked bread.

WHITING

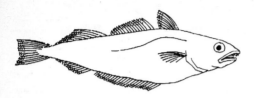

Another fish with a history and so under-estimated today.
The whiting, rolled and curled in days gone by, was sold to
feed the 'downstairs' staff at the big house — many a Duke
and Earl would appreciate his fish pie made with this
cousin of the cod family. A little on the dry side, poaching,
cooking in a parcel, or adding a little white wine, all help to
keep the fish moist.

Fried Whiting with Cucumber Cream

Serves 4

Ingredients

	Metric	Imperial	American
little oil or butter for frying			
fillets of fresh whiting, tossed in seasoned flour	4	4	4
butter	25 g	1 oz	2 tbsp
cucumber, peeled and finely sliced	½	½	½
juice of lemon	1	1	1
fromage frais	150 ml	¼ pint	⅔ cup
seasoning to taste			

Method

Heat a little oil or butter in a frying pan, fry the fish for 2 minutes each side. During this time heat the butter in a saucepan, add the cucumber and simmer for 4 minutes. Add the lemon juice and stir in the fromage frais. Season to taste, pour the sauce over the fish and serve.

WINKLES

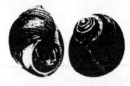

Great fun if you have loads of patience. A tiny mollusc packed tightly into a round shell, determined to be picked out with a pin. Look out for the seafood stalls when around London on a Sunday stroll — or try Brighton Pier. Do not under-estimate this little mite — it is packed full of all the minerals that will enhance your love life. The saying reads 'the amorous prawn' — try a winkle!

WITCH

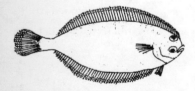

Cook as for Flounder or Plaice. Sometimes known as a Torbay sole and a witch flounder — never mind the name, this fish 'spells' tasty, nutritional eating.

Index

aïoli, 19
anchovies, 22
  anchovy and potato
  pie, 23
angler fish *see* monkfish
apple mayonnaise, 27-8
Arbroath smokies, 24

bass *see* sea bass
blackjack *see* coley
bloater, 25
  bloater paste, 26
brandy dressing for fresh
  lobster, 80
bream/sea bream, 26
  grilled bream, 26-7
brill, 27
  steamed brill fillets with
  apple mayonnaise, 27-
8
brown shrimps *see* shrimps
buckling, 28

carp, 29
  boiled carp, 29-30
catfish, 30-31
chicken turbot *see* turbot
clams, 32
  clams with pasta
  shells, 32-3
coalfish *see* coley
cockles, 33
cod, 35
  salt cod with
  tomatoes, 36
  simple cod bake with
  mushrooms, 35-6
cod's roe
  cod roe fritters, 37
  smoked cod's roe, 38
coley, 38
  cheap and cheerful
  fish pie, 38-9
conger eel, 40
  microwave conger
  casserole, 40-41
crab, 41-3

crab tea for two, 43
Cromer crab, 44
spider crab soup, 44-5
velvet crab, 45
crawfish au natural for
  two, 46
crayfish, 46-7
  crayfish the
  Scandinavian way, 47
Cromer crab *see under* crab
cuttlefish, 47

dab, 48
  fried dabs for
  breakfast, 48-9
DHA (docosahexaenoic
  acid), 9
dogfish *see* huss
dory *see* John Dory
Dover sole, 49-50
  grilled sole, 50
Dublin Bay
  prawns, 50-51
  scampi in a basket, 52

eels, 53
  jellied eels, 53
  slimming with eels, 54
  see also conger eel
elvers, 55
EPA (eicosapentaenoic
  acid), 9

fenugreek special, the
  Shirly, 80-81
Finnan haddock, 56-8
  cullen skink, 57-8
  Finnan haddock for
  breakfast, 56-7
flake *see* huss
flounder (fluke), 58
  witch flounder *see* witch
freezing, 14

garfish, 59
grey mullet, 59
  baked grey mullet, 60
gurnard, 60

haddock, 61
  fish and chips, 62
  smoked haddock
  soufflé, 63-4

smokie and hot
  potato, 24
  see also Finnan haddock
hake, 64
  creamy hake bake, 65
halibut, 65-6
  halibut steaks with
  lemon sauce, 66
herbs, 15
herring, 67-8
  marinated herring, 69
  soused herring, 69-70
  Welsh herring pie, 68
herring roe, 69
hollandaise sauce, 19
huss, 70-71

John Dory, 72
  poached John Dory, 73

king scallops *see*
  queenies; scallops
kippers, 74
  kippers in a jug for
  breakfast, 74
  poor man's smoked
  salmon, 75

lemon sole, 76
  Devon lemon sole with
  fresh orange,76-7
ling, 77
  Good Friday pie with
  mushy peas, 78
lobster, 79-80
  brandy dressing for
  fresh lobster, 80
  grilled lobster, 81
  how to prepare
  lobster, 82
  the Shirly fenugreek
  special, 80-81

mackerel, 83
  grilled very fresh
  mackerel, 83-4
  smoked mackerel
  pâté, 84
mayonnaise
  aïoli, 19
  apple, 27-8
  brandy dressing for
  fresh lobster, 80

poached trout with tangy mayonnaise, 117-18
the Shirly fenugreek special, 80-81
megrim, 84
monkfish, 85
monkfish and garlic, 85-6
mullet *see* grey mullet; red mullet
mussels, 86-7
barbecued farmed mussels, 88
boiled mussels with garlic and wine (moules à la Marinière), 87-8
simple mussel salad, 89

oysters, 90-93, 95
frozen oysters on beds of spinach, 93

peas, Good Friday pie with mushy, 78
pies
anchovy and potato pie, 23
cheap and cheerful fish pie, 38-9
Good Friday pie with mushy peas, 78
Stargazy pie, 96
Welsh herring pie, 68
woof pie from Yorkshire, 31-2
pike, 95
pilchards, 95
stargazy pie, 96
plaice, 96
pollack, 96-7
pollack with mustard sauce, 97
porbeagle, 110
prawns, 97-8
prawn cocktail, 98-9
see also Dublin Bay Prawns
princess scallops, *see* queenies; scallops

queenies in fromage frais sauce, 100
quenelles, 95

ray, 101
red mullet, 101-2
red mullet in a parcel, 102
rice, tuna with brown, 121
rigg *see* huss
rock salmon *see* catfish
rock *see* huss
rockfish, 31
roe *see* cod's roe; herring roe

saffron, 15
saffron squid, 115
saithe *see* coley
salads
simple mussel salad, 89
tuna salad for one, 120
salmon, 103-4
baked salmon, 104-5
smoked salmon, 105-6
salmon trout, 106
salt cod, *see under* cod
sardines, 106-7
sauces
fromage frais, 100
hollandaise, 19
lemon, 17-18, 66
minty cream, 18
mustard, 97
parsley, 18
scallops, 107
scampi, 50-51
scampi in a basket, 52
sea bass, 108
baked sea bass for a party, 108-9
sea bream *see* bream
sea trout, 118
sea urchins, 109
sea vegetables (seaweed), 14-15
shark, 110
shrimps, 110-11
pink, 111

skate, 111
fried skate wings with fresh lemon, 112
skate knob kebabs, 112
smelts, 112
smoked haddock soufflé, 63-4
smoked mackerel pâté, 84
smoked trout, 119
smokies, Arbroath, 24
smokie and hot potato, 24
sole *see* Dover sole, lemon sole
sole, Torbay *see* witch
soup
fish soup, 20-21
spider crab soup, 44-5
sprats, Vera's fried, 113
squid, 113-14
fritto misto to cook at home, 114
saffron squid, 115

tope, 110, 116
trout, 116-17
fisherman's trout, 118
poached trout with tangy mayonnaise, 117-18
salmon trout, 106
sea trout, 106, 118
smoked trout, 119
tuna, 119
tuna mousse, 119-120
tuna salad for one, 120
tuna with brown rice, 121
turbot, 122

velvet crab, 45

whelks, 123
whitebait, 123-4
oven cooked, 124
whiting, 125
fried whiting with cucumber cream, 125-6
winkles, 126
witch, 126
wolf fish, 31
woof pie, 31-2